Further praise for Wendy Ha

"Wendy Harpham is an inspiration to all touched by cancer. Her solid advice and upbeat perspective are invaluable."
—Diane Blum, M.S.W., executive director, Cancer Care, Inc.

"If a newly diagnosed person reads one book about cancer, *Diagnosis: Cancer* is the one it should be. It is a guide through the maze of uncertainty and a way to begin taking control over the crisis of cancer. For the survivor finished with treatment, it answers nagging questions and updates the knowledge that is critical to dealing with a life-altering experience."
—Joan F. Hermann, L.S.W., director, Social Work Services, Fox Chase Cancer Center

"The new edition of *Diagnosis: Cancer* is an important resource for newly diagnosed cancer patients and their families. Dr. Harpham approaches this complicated topic from an unusual vantage point— that of both physician and patient. This lucidly written and informative book is loaded with practical information and sage advice. Highly recommended to patients, families, and physicians caring for cancer patients. Each group will find it to be of great value."
—Marvin J. Stone, M.D., M.A.C.P., chief of oncology, director, Baylor Charles A. Sammons Cancer Center

"In this much-expanded edition, Dr. Harpham encourages people with cancer to develop a partnership with members of the cancer care team, gives readers access to 'state-of-the-art' information, and provides a thorough and balanced discussion about alternative treatments. As a nurse, I know that accurate and timely information allays unnecessary fears and gives people what they need to know to advocate for good, quality cancer care. *Diagnosis: Cancer* is a readable and easy-to-understand resource for people facing cancer."
—Pamela J. Haylock, R.N., M.A., president, Oncology Nursing Society

"When a diagnosis of cancer raises endless questions for patients and their families, Dr. Wendy Harpham—herself a cancer survivor who has been through it all—provides clear, simple but comprehensive and compassionate answers and explanations to ease their concerns and help them make the best possible decisions about everything from choosing treatments to coping with feelings, family and friends. This book—the very best of its kind—should be a bible for everyone facing cancer."
—Jane E. Brody, personal health columnist, *New York Times*

"The diagnosis of cancer is frightening to anyone. The newly diagnosed patient is really interested in only one thing—becoming a long-term cancer survivor. This book, *Diagnosis: Cancer*, is the road map for the patient wishing to make the journey from victim to survivor. Dr. Harpham, a cancer survivor herself, provides practical, understandable, and reliable information for this journey. The questions asked and answered are well researched, pertinent, and up to the minute. Advice from the seemingly mundane like 'Is cancer contagious?' to the latest advice on experimental therapies are all included. If you take one book with you on your journey when you or a loved one is faced with the diagnosis of cancer, this is the one. It's the atlas to good decision making and survivorship."

—Leonard A. Zwelling, M.D., M.B.A., vice president for research administration, University of Texas M.D. Anderson Cancer Center

"Recommended for every newly diagnosed cancer patient. Most new patients have two factors in common: fear of the unknown and no idea of what questions to ask. This book clearly solves both problems with readily understandable, easy to read, compassionate explanations."

—Richard A. Bloch, author (with Annette Bloch) of *Fighting Cancer* and founder of the R. A. Bloch Cancer Foundation

"No one writes better about cancer than Wendy Schlessel Harpham, M.D. Her gifts as a doctor inform every page of this sensitive, knowledgeable, and practical guide. Because she is a cancer survivor, Dr. Harpham has a unique perspective, and with wonderful clarity and down-to-earth wisdom she covers every single aspect of a cancer diagnosis. She made my own cancer journey not only easier, but, yes, more interesting."

—Natalie Robins, author of *The Girl Who Died Twice* and the Living with Cancer series published in *Self* magazine

"The first few months after the diagnosis of cancer are made even more difficult because you are in a new world with many unfamiliar people, rules, and questions to be answered. Wendy Schlessel Harpham, M.D., in her book *Diagnosis: Cancer*, sets forth an enormous amount of practical information which, I am sure, will alleviate much of the uncertainty and anxiety that is part of the new surroundings. I believe that reducing that stress will improve the quality of life and may have a positive effect on the course of the illness."

—Harold H. Benjamin, Ph.D., founder, The Wellness Community

Diagnosis:
CANCER

Also by Wendy Schlessel Harpham, M.D.

After Cancer: A Guide to Your New Life

When a Parent Has Cancer: A Guide to Caring for Your Children
with the illustrated children's book, *Becky and the Worry Cup*

The Hope Tree: Kids Talk About Breast Cancer
(coauthor with Laura Numeroff)

Diagnosis:
CANCER

YOUR GUIDE

TO THE FIRST MONTHS

OF HEALTHY SURVIVORSHIP

EXPANDED AND UPDATED

Wendy Schlessel Harpham, M.D.

W. W. Norton & Company

New York   London

Manufacturing by The Haddon Craftsmen, Inc.
Production manager: Amanda Morrison

Library of Congress Cataloging-in-Publication Data

Harpham, Wendy Schlessel.
Diagnosis, cancer : your guide to the first months of healthy survivorship /
Wendy Schlessel Harpham ; illustrations by Ann Bliss Pilcher. — Updated
and expanded.
      p. cm.
Revised and updated ed. published with subtitle: Your guide through the first
few months.
Includes bibliographical references and index.
    ISBN 0-393-32460-5 (pbk.)
 1. Cancer—Popular works.   2. Cancer—Psychological aspects.   I. Title.
    RC263.H36 2003
    616.99'4—dc21

                                                        2002156597

W. W. Norton & Company, Inc.
500 Fifth Avenue, New York, N.Y. 10110
www.wwnorton.com

W. W. Norton & Company Ltd.
Castle House, 75/76 Wells Street, London W1T 3QT

1 2 3 4 5 6 7 8 9 0

Dedication

—

To Brenda Casey, R.N., John H. Cottey, M.D.,
Susan M. Creagan, M.D., David G. Maloney, M.D.,
Lizanne Piercy, M.D., and James F. Strauss, M.D.

To the families of Congregation Beth Torah and
Presbyterian Hospital of Dallas who helped us

To Ted, Rebecca, Jessica, and William

Our knowledge about cancer is constantly changing. This book is not intended as a substitute for competent medical care. It serves to supplement the information provided by your doctors and nurses.

Contents

Prologue

I saw it all: injuries and illnesses, medical disasters and miracles. As a doctor of internal medicine, I was acutely aware of the fragility and capriciousness of life, and appreciated my health and good fortune. Caring for patients in my solo practice was demanding, rewarding, and the perfect way to express my gratitude. Each day, after finishing with my last patient, I'd shift gears and eagerly rush home to join my husband, Ted, in caring for our three lively children all under six years old. Life was good, and I knew it.

Just before Thanksgiving 1990, enlarging lymph nodes in my groin caused excruciating pain in my leg and back, and landed me in my own hospital. Two surgeries revealed a stage 3 indolent non-Hodgkin's lymphoma (a type of cancer with no known cure) and yanked me across the great divide from physician to patient. In all my years of doctoring I'd never felt as if my white coat protected me in some magical way, yet being told I had cancer was shocking.

Mine wasn't the typical "new patient" experience. For me, the sterile hospital was reassuringly familiar turf. The oncologist who was called in to consult on my case was a longtime colleague whom I respected and trusted completely. From the start, I understood what all my doctors and nurses were doing and why, and I could communicate with them in technical medical language. The downside of being a physician-patient was that I knew too much. I'd seen too much. Graphic memories of past patients deprived me of the comfort and strength born of innocence and denial. The numbing shock, primal fear, and childlike helplessness and dependency stretched each of those first days into what seemed like a week. Accustomed to handling my patients' life-and-death crises with professional calm, I was blindsided by the magnitude of my fear, anxiety, disorientation, and sadness when I was the patient.

In the midst of these intense emotions, one fact grounded me and became my main mantra to this day: *I can't always choose my circumstances, but I can choose how I deal with them.* I vowed to bring everything I knew and all the strength I could muster to becoming an effective patient. Easier said than done. After years of teaching my patients to call me when they developed signs and symptoms of potential problems, I found myself hesitating to report my fatigue at my checkups or call my doctors at midnight when I developed a fever. Self-consciousness, embarrassment, insecurity, anxiety, and fear made it hard for me to do what I knew to be the right thing.

The disciplined doctor in me governed my actions and overrode any reluctance. It's a good thing, too, because during the months of my intensive chemotherapy a number of complications developed, some of which required hospitalization. The important point is not that I had complications but that the problems were nipped in the bud. Each hospitalization lasted only one to three days because of both my willingness to call my doctors with early signs of problems and their responsiveness and expertise.

Accepting my role as patient wasn't too hard because I knew that doing so would help me get better. Hanging up my white coat and stethoscope was another story. After my diagnosis, the doctors with whom I shared weekend "call" cared for my patients while I used precious time and energy trying unsuccessfully to arrange a substitute physician for my patients. When I ended up closing my practice temporarily, a small group of friends and family came to my home to stuff two thousand "Dear Patient" letters. Mailing that stack of letters was an especially painful loss in the string of losses that began in the emergency room four weeks earlier. Everyone laughed when my five-year-old daughter responded to a comment about her mother being a doctor by saying, "Well, my mommy *used* to be a doctor!" I chuckled, too, sadly.

Hoping to find the good in something awful, I dusted off my violin and warmed up on a few easy études. In the ten years since I'd last opened my violin case, I'd often daydreamed about playing, never doubting that when my kids were grown I would find time again. Suddenly, I had too much time on my hands. Making music was one of my first escapes from cancer. Improving my violin playing was one of my first goals unrelated to cancer. Realizing that I could still do things that I enjoyed was one of my first steps toward renewed wholeness after cancer.

Practicing my violin soon became my break not only from cancer but also from writing. You see, as I found ways to ease my own physical and emotional discomforts, or at least better understand them, I felt compelled to share what I was learning. I'm a doctor; helping people is what I do. How else can I explain why, during the months of my initial chemotherapy, I devoted time and energy to creating a pamphlet of information and advice to help other patients with cancer?

To be honest, my motives were not *all* altruistic. During the earliest weeks of my illness, I had discovered that writing distracted me from my leg and back pain, my chronic nausea (a common problem in that pre-Zofran® era), and my loneliness during the periods of isolation that were necessary during the days when my blood counts dipped dangerously low (another common problem in that pre-Neupogen® era). Tapping away at the computer keys drowned out the terrifying thoughts running amok in my head. Just as important, doing something for patients helped me hold on to my identity as a doctor.

Writing a pamphlet proved to be the perfect project. I completed it just as I finished my chemotherapy. The only problem was this: Weighing in at over 120 pages, it wasn't a pamphlet anymore. It was a full-fledged book. I've been writing ever since. I can't finish one project before another engages my attention. During the preparation of *After Cancer* and *When a Parent Has Cancer*, I delved into issues discussed only briefly in *Diagnosis: Cancer*. Not surprisingly, I learned a lot in the process and found myself thinking, "If only I knew then what I know now." New philosophies and mantras that became second nature would have been helpful in the earliest stages of my survivorship. Fortunately, in 1998, I could include them in the revised version of *Diagnosis: Cancer,* a project prompted by the need to update the medical information.

Had I been cured after my first or second or, even, third round of treatment, I undoubtedly would have returned to clinical medicine and let my writing career and cancer history fade into the background. But, I wasn't cured. Almost annually, my lymphoma recurred, forcing me to grapple over and over with two essential questions: How do I get the best care? How do I live as fully as possible while going through treatment?

Recurrence, radiation therapy, immunotherapy, investigational therapy, chronic aftereffects, late effects, and long-term survival are no longer just academic topics. All have become part of my personal survivorship. Issues that I thought I'd addressed during my first round of chemotherapy looked different each time I was faced with another diagnosis of lymphoma. I've looked at alternative therapies and clinical trials with the mind of a scientist and the heart of a patient desperate to survive. Problems with loss, uncertainty, and lack of control kept resurfacing, forcing me to rethink them again and again, and encouraging me to find new and better ways of living with these unavoidable realities of survivorship.

My choices, hopes, and expectations have changed over the years as science has made progress in the diagnosis and treatment of cancer. This current remission, my seventh and longest by far—the result of FDA-approved Rituxan®, a drug that wasn't available when I was first diagnosed—gives new meaning to my oldest mantra, "There is always hope."

My evolution as a survivor also reflects the experiences of people whose paths have intersected mine. Advocacy work and public speaking have connected me with people from all over North America who are dealing with cancer, personally or professionally. The tiresome inconveniences of traveling have been offset by my fun hobby: searching for a commemorative thimble from each new city in which I do survivorship work. As my thimble collection has grown, so has my understanding of survivorship. I've mulled over the questions, vignettes, and insights tendered by hundreds of patients, friends and family members, and professionals in oncology. Each week, it seems, I've modified some philosophy or found stronger, clearer language for conveying a feeling or conclusion.

This edition of *Diagnosis: Cancer* is the result of my marathon exploration. I've kept the order and tone of most of the questions exactly the same as in the first edition, trusting the value to readers of the perspective I held in the weeks and months following my diagnosis. I can never again capture the aura of a first diagnosis. Cancer has become too familiar, too normal. The novelty, confusion, and untamed fear are long gone. This loss is why, now, I can bring something more to a book for newly diagnosed patients: a long-term perspective on those first few months. My current beliefs about what people need to know, and what philosophies and handles might help have withstood the test of time.

I don't believe there's one "right" way to deal with cancer. You need to find the best way *for you*. This book is premised on the conviction that your medical outcome is determined by more than just your diagnosis and prognosis. What happens is the end result of all the factors that influence your body's response to disease such as your cancer treatments, nutrition, physical activity, spirituality, will to live, genes, support, love, luck, attitude, expectations, and hope. What constitutes *your* healing balance is unique and dynamic, changing as your situation changes and as you change.

How do you tip the healing balance in your favor? I wish I had magic dust—a sprinkling that would make your cancer disappear, and with it all the problems in its wake. But, I don't. So, I continue with the work that has been my life mission: helping others through the synergy of science and caring. More than ever before, science offers patients something that is unique and invaluable. You can't underestimate the importance of choosing the cancer treatment that gives you the best chance. At the same time, much about the body's ability to survive cancer remains mysterious and responsive to the healing forces of caring.

Years ago, I outlived the prognosis given me when I was first diagnosed. Twice, I tried going back to clinical medicine. Both times, illness and the need for further cancer treatment forced me to stop. Since then, I've yet to regain the stamina needed for direct patient care. Accepting my limits, I've taken another route to fulfilling my mission: writing. Every morning, I work on an article, book, or lecture that dissects survivorship into digestible morsels of sound information and reality-based hope. Every afternoon, I rest. Years ago, I awoke from one of my afternoon naps with an idea for a novel having nothing to do with cancer. I quickly scribbled down notes for a story line, anticipating the day when my books on cancer are found only on dusty shelves alongside books on iron lungs.

Some people wonder why I don't work on my novel now, especially since my own illness, thankfully, has finally faded into the background of my life. I often forget when my next checkup is due or the exact dates of my recurrences, and yet my writing remains focused on survivorship. It's not a fear of fiction but that I remember how hard it was when I was first diagnosed. Even with all my advantages—my loving husband, a caring health-care team, good health insurance, medical knowledge, spiritual faith, and family and community support—it was a tough time. I feel obligated to use my perspective as physician-survivor to try to make it a bit easier, safer, and less frightening for others.

You don't have to be a doctor to get good health care. When you can sort through the information overload, take advantage of advances in science and technology, and communicate well with your health-care team, you can make wise decisions. Writing *Diagnosis: Cancer* is one way that I can encourage you to benefit from both science and caring and create your own unique healing balance. My life's mission hasn't changed since medical school, just the venue.

A sense of obligation isn't the only reason I keep writing about survivorship. This work is how I express my gratitude for my health and good fortune. I do it to honor the people who have helped me. And, I do it for me. Today, good nutrition, regular exercise, prayer, daily rest, violin duets with my son, lots of hugs, love and friendship, girls' high-school volleyball, occasional back massages, commemorative thimbles and the possibility of collecting ones from all fifty states, laughter, and writing for patients while I am surrounded by the bright pink walls and grape purple doors of my study are some of the elements of *my* healing balance.

Until reliable, nontoxic cures and preventive measures are available for every type of cancer, I'll keep writing for survivors and their families, as well as the health-care professionals who care for them. I'll keep traveling, adding thimbles to my collection to remind me of the people I meet and the insights I gain. I'll keep revising *Diagnosis: Cancer* until the words "You have cancer" no longer elicit fear, for they no longer pose a threat. And, one day, I'll start my novel.

With hope, Wendy

Acknowledgments to the Third Edition

I'll always be indebted to my friends and colleagues who offered literary feedback and emotional support during the writing of the first and second editions of *Diagnosis: Cancer*. For this third edition, I want to extend my thanks to my oncologist, James F. Strauss, M.D., for our ongoing medical discussions and his review of the medical chapters, as well as his genuine interest in all my writing. I also thank Lori A. Kunkel, M.D., David G. Maloney, M.D., and Gabriel A. Shapiro, M.D., for their feedback on specific medical questions and sections, and Debra Sue Bruck, Brenda S. Casey, R.N., Barbara Hoffman, J.D., and Adele M. O'Reilly for their time and input.

Special thanks to Mary Cunnane, the editor at W. W. Norton who offered me a contract for the first edition twenty-four hours after receiving the manuscript. When Mary moved, I was fortunate to have my book inherited by Amy Cherry, an editor who shares my hope of helping others through words. I appreciate Amy's commitment to keeping *Diagnosis: Cancer* updated and available to survivors.

I am grateful for my three children: Rebecca, Jessica, and William. With generosity that makes me proud, they have given me the time and space I've needed to work on this book. Lastly, I thank my husband, Ted. He's my harshest critic and my greatest fan. His uncensored feedback makes my books better; his love makes me better.

Introduction

——

From the time of discovery and for the balance of life, an individual diagnosed with cancer is a *survivor.*
    —National Coalition for Cancer Survivorship

A *survivor* who gets good care and lives as fully as possible is a *Healthy Survivor.* —Wendy S. Harpham, M.D.

You have just been told that you have cancer. You are a cancer survivor. Your world has come to a sudden stop whether you are young or old, recovering from a simple biopsy or a complex surgery, feeling sick or perfectly healthy, enjoying fruitful times or struggling with problems at work and home. Life is not going to be the way you planned, at least not for the immediate future. You may feel overwhelmed with information, emotions, and responsibilities that make it hard to think clearly. Yet, important decisions need to be made right now about your medical evaluation and treatment, and your situation at work, school, and home.

This book will help you and your family get through these first few months as easily and safely as possible. It will teach you how to ask the right questions, and make the best decisions *for you* from day one. The philosophy behind this book is that you did not choose to have cancer, but you can determine how you deal with it. You can decide to be a Healthy Survivor, by which I mean you get the best medical care possible *and* you minimize the pain, debility, and loss due to your illness. As a Healthy Survivor, every day you take steps to maximize your chances of recovery *and* optimize your quality of life.

To say "Knowledge is power" is trite, but true, when it comes to cancer. Sound knowledge enables you to participate in your care and be your own best advocate. At the very least, you will understand what is happening, even when you prefer to leave all decision making to others. Knowledge will help you regain some control, lessen fear and pain, and look toward your future in a hopeful and productive way.

Based on my experiences as a physician and long-term cancer survivor, this book offers information and advice for dealing with the medical, practical, and emotional aspects of survivorship. Not all the recommendations will apply to you since this book covers the wide variety of newly diagnosed cancer patients, and you and your situation are unique. In this book, I use the word "family" to refer to all those people who care for you. Your family may include children, parents, siblings, a spouse, a companion, a lover, close friends and colleagues, and other associates. The key is that these people are involved in your life and are affected by what is happening to you.

Each chapter contains bold-print questions followed by brief answers or outlines of how you can get the best answer(s) for you. Statements that can be used as helpful reminders or inspirational handles are boldfaced. Each topic is addressed more fully in books available at your local bookstores and libraries, and in pamphlets, videos, Web casts, and reputable Web sites made available by local and national cancer organizations.

The appendixes include tips for being an effective patient, a glossary of medical terms defined in lay language (these terms appear in boldface type in the text), a brief resource list, a sample medication sheet, an explanation of common medical tests, and an explanation of medical abbreviations.

You and your family members can read this book cover to cover, using whatever information you find helpful. Or, you can skim the questions and index for topics that interest you now and leave the other sections to read when the topics apply to you more directly or when you feel better equipped to review them. Keep this book handy so that you can reread it periodically and refer to it as needed over the next few months. Many survivors find that the same information and advice help in different ways as they go through the various phases of diagnosis, evaluation, treatment, and recovery.

You are not alone. More than one million Americans are diagnosed with cancer each year. One out of every three women and one out of every two men will be diagnosed with cancer sometime in their life. There are almost nine million cancer survivors in America. You can learn from veteran survivors how to get through the first few months without having to discover everything for yourself.

Remember:

- Learn as much or as little as you are ready to at this time. You do not need to learn or understand everything right away.
- If you do not understand something, keep asking! Many different resources can help you get the answers you seek, and many people are available who want to help you get your answers.
- You are an individual. Your cancer and your situation are unique. Find out about your cancer, and learn what you can do to become a Healthy Survivor.
- The treatments for cancer are improving all the time. Cancer treatments continue to become safer and more effective, and new research is beginning to yield treatments that are less toxic. New and better ways are available to prevent, minimize, and treat side effects. Don't let fear of treatment keep you from getting evaluated or treated.
- We are talking about *your life*. Right now, nothing is as important as finding out about your cancer, and making wise decisions about how to treat it.

It's time to begin the road to Healthy Survivorship. The first step is to learn the basics about cancer in chapter 1.

Diagnosis:

CANCER

———

1

Understanding Your Diagnosis

After finding out that you have cancer, you may want to "get the show on the road" and start treatment. Meanwhile, your physicians may be recommending more tests, and family and friends may be uging you to get a second opinion. The first step to getting better is making as accurate a diagnosis as possible and determining how your cancer is behaving in your body. "Haste makes waste" is an adage that may help calm any sense of urgency you might be feeling.

Take the time necessary to learn about your disease and treatment options, and to make the best decisions with your doctors. Why? With some types of cancer, your first shot at cure is your best one, although not necessarily the only one. Some treatments preclude the use of others down the line. You don't want to rush into just any treatment. Also, your physicians need to know about the health of all your organs so that they can prevent or minimize treatment-related problems when possible. They need time to learn about your cancer and the physical condition of your body.

You may not want to take the time and energy to learn a lot about your cancer right now. You may not see the necessity in a similar way that you don't study transmission repair when a car mechanic informs you that your transmission needs work. Or, you may see the value but feel squeezed for time as you try to take care of work or home responsibilities in between your doctor visits, tests, and procedures. You may find it too upsetting and just prefer to wait until things quiet down.

The problem with this approach is that life won't quiet down until some critical decisions have been made by you with your doctors. A basic understanding of the language and medicine of cancer will help you understand what is going on and participate in your care to whatever degree you feel most comfortable. You don't have to learn everything; you just need to know *enough* to talk with your doctors and help them make the best decisions for you.

Your doctors will tell you if you need treatment urgently. You may not have the luxury of time to learn all about your cancer and obtain second opinions before starting treatment. For some newly diagnosed patients, waiting even a few hours or days increases the risk of a poor outcome and may actually cause them to lose a small window of opportunity for cure or improvement. If your doctors feel that treatment is needed immediately to prevent serious complications or preserve the possibility of cure, they will complete the evaluation while you are receiving your first treatments. Although it can be more frightening when everything happens so fast, your situation may make "Treat now, learn later" the best approach for you. Oncologists are trained to judge how quickly treatment needs to be started to give you the best outcome. This chapter will discuss a methodical approach to the evaluation of your cancer, and assumes that you have time to do this safely before beginning treatment.

What is cancer?

Cancer is a very *general term* that refers to hundreds of *different* diseases. All types of cancer

- have uncontrolled growth of abnormal **cells**;
- can spread through the blood and **lymph** (a clear fluid that circulates in the body) to other parts of the body.

Each type of cancer is a different disease. For example, breast cancer is a different disease than colon cancer. In addition, progress in the diagnosis of cancer has revealed that each type of cancer may be made up of a variety of different cancers. For instance, some breast cancers have one set of genetic abnormalities and behave in one general way while other breast cancers have different abnormalities and tend to behave in another way.

Only by learning about *your* specific type of cancer can you understand your situation. Your cancer may be slow-growing and expected to cause you few, if any, problems for a long time. Your cancer may be fast-growing (aggressive) and most assuredly will cause serious problems if not treated immediately. Your cancer may be curable with today's therapies. Or, your cancer may be treatable but rarely curable with current standard therapies. Your cancer may be expected to spread to other parts of your body, such as the bones, brain, or lungs. Or, you may have the type of cancer that rarely spreads or only spreads late in the course of illness. These distinctions are important because each type of cancer needs a different treatment.

Am I going to die?

Cancer is an illness, not a death sentence. There are estimated to be almost nine million cancer survivors in America, most of whom were diagnosed over five years ago (and most of these survivors are considered cured). Many cancers are not curable but are still treatable, allowing the person to live a relatively normal life much like someone with a **chronic** illness such as diabetes. Rarely, a person's cancer will disappear completely without any treatment (a "**spontaneous remission**"). *Without treatment,* the usual course of events is that cancer continues to grow, eventually blocking the body's normal functions and causing death.

Am I going to have pain?

Pain is one of the most dreaded and common symptoms associated with cancer. It doesn't have to be. Most people with cancer have no pain when the cancer is early; fewer than half of newly diagnosed patients have pain. When cancer pain occurs, 85 percent of patients find relief with simple pain pills. For the remaining 15 percent, effective therapies are available and most patients can achieve excellent pain control. Pain is an important symptom to address because it affects your quality of life and state of mind, *and* it is treatable. Keep your doctors informed about any pain, even mild pain, so that you can work together to achieve optimum pain control (see the section on pain control, pages 107–17).

What is my diagnosis? What type of cancer do I have?

Your **diagnosis** is the name of your illness, in this case the name of your cancer. The only way to make a definite diagnosis of cancer is by doing a **biopsy** (getting a piece of suspicious tissue) and examining it. A specialized doctor, or **pathologist**, often can determine what kind of cancer you have by how the cells look under the microscope. Lung cancer cells look like lung cells but are changed in ways that are characteristic of cancer. As an analogy, if your next-door neighbor is enraged, you can still recognize your neighbor even though he looks different with an angry facial expression. Pathologists also perform sophisticated tests on the cancer cells to help determine the cells' place of origin.

The name of a cancer is based on where it first started, if this can be determined. Cancer in the lung that *started in the lung* is lung cancer. Cancer in the lung that *started in the breast* is breast cancer now situated in the lung. If you have lung cancer that has spread to your bones, the cancer cells in your bones look the same as the cancer cells in your lung.

Your cancer may fall into one of the following types, in decreasing order of incidence:

Carcinoma—cancer that started in "epithelial tissue" (skin; secreting portion of glands and ducts; certain sense organs; and the lining and covering tissues of organs, cavities, and tubes)
Lymphoma—cancer that started in the lymph system (**lymph nodes, spleen, lymphatic** vessels)
Leukemia—cancer that started in the white blood cells in the **bone marrow**

Multiple myeloma—cancer that started in the plasma cells in the bone marrow

Sarcoma—cancer that started in the bone or soft tissue (muscles, nerves, tendons, blood vessels)

Your cancer may be one that doesn't fall neatly into one of these categories, such as glioma (of brain), melanoma (of skin), and germ cell tumors.

What are hematopoietic cancers?

Leukemia, lymphoma, and myeloma are hematopoietic cancers. These cancers start in a blood-forming organ, such as the bone marrow, lymph nodes, or, rarely, spleen. Since normal cells from the bone marrow and lymph nodes circulate throughout the body, **malignant** cells of hematopoietic cancers can circulate throughout the body.

What are "solid" cancers?

In contrast to the bone marrow and lymph nodes, organs such as the liver, lung, brain, muscle, breast, colon, and prostate are considered solid organs. Normally, cells from these organs are not found in the circulation. Cancers that start in these organs are called "solid cancers" or "solid tumors."

Why is my diagnosis so important?

Since each type of cancer is really a separate disease, your diagnosis needs to be as accurate as possible so that you get treated for the right disease. Your diagnosis is a key factor in determining your prognosis and treatment options.

Are there any differences between a lesion, tumor, neoplasm, malignancy, and cancer?

The words **lesion, tumor, neoplasm, malignancy,** and cancer are often used interchangeably even though they have different definitions. Be sure you know exactly what the user means.

A lesion is an abnormal area, benign or malignant. Mouth ulcers and bruises on your arms may be referred to as lesions.

When physicians know that bumps on your skin are little areas of cancer, they may refer to these areas of cancer as "lesions."

A tumor is any abnormal swelling or enlargement. A tumor can be due to infection, bleeding, cancer, or anything else that causes an area of swelling. When physicians *know* that spots in your lung are cancer, they may refer to your cancer as tumors, as in "Your tumors are responding to the treatment."

A neoplasm is any overgrowth of cells, benign (not cancer) or malignant (cancer). **Benign** skin tags and malignant skin cancer are both neoplasms.

"Benign," when used to describe a tumor or sample of tissue, is a descriptive term that means "not cancer." A benign growth cannot spread through the blood or lymph to other parts of the body. It can cause serious problems if it grows near a vital structure, but benign growths are rarely life-threatening. Skin tags and uterine fibroids are examples of benign growths. Technically speaking, there is no such thing as a benign cancer.

"Malignant" is a descriptive word that means "cancerous." All cancers are malignant. When microscopic evaluation of tissue reveals evidence of malignancy, it is cancer. Malignant tumors can invade surrounding tissues and spread (metastasize) to other sites.

In summary:

Lesion = abnormal area = benign or malignant
Tumor = swelling or enlargement = benign or malignant
Neoplasm = abnormal growth = benign or malignant
Benign = *not* cancer, *not* malignant
Malignant = cancer

Is there any uncertainty about my diagnosis?

Usually your diagnosis is definite, and no matter how many different doctors read your biopsy slides, they will all agree as to the specific type of cancer that you have. Determining the type and malignant nature of a tumor is not an exact science, and sometimes the diagnosis is not certain even when all the tests are done perfectly. For example, your doctors may know that you have a carcinoma, but can't tell what kind—breast, lung, whatever. The uncertainty remains because of the characteristics of your particular cancer cells. When the specific diagnosis is at all unclear, your slides and test results should be reviewed by several doctors, one of whom preferably has special expertise in your general type of cancer or in cancers of unknown origin.

What is my prognosis?

Prognosis is the estimation of how you will do (such as the course of your illness, your chance for recovery, and how your disease will end). Your prognosis depends on

- your type of cancer;
- how aggressive your cancer is (see next question);
- how far advanced your cancer is (see "Staging," page 23);
- your age and physical fitness;
- the presence or absence of any other medical conditions;
- many factors that cannot be measured, such as your will to live.

Nobody on earth can foretell your future. Your prognosis is not a fact but an educated guess based on statistics derived from a large group of people in the past whose cancer situation shared similarities with yours. Your prognosis is a vital piece of information that helps to determine the best treatment plan for you. It provides one way to understand how serious your immediate and long-term situation is, which helps you and your family prepare for whatever lies ahead.

It is impossible to predict exactly how *you* will do because you are unique. There are no statistics for a large group of people of the exact same age as you, with precisely the same amount of cancer as you, in exactly the same overall health, receiving the exact same treatments, and having the exact same lifestyle, luck, will to live, and so on.

Another reason why precise predictions can't be made is that new treatments that are safer and/or more effective become available regularly. Because the newer therapies being used today have only been given to patients for a relatively short time, long-range information about these treatments won't be obtainable for many years. In other words, the prognosis you get today does not reflect the improvement in prognosis that your current therapy may provide over older therapies. In addition, your prognosis does not take into account promising new therapies currently under investigation that will prove to be more effective and that will become available to you in the future.

The statistics that help determine your prognosis are based on the best information that doctors have today, but they are limited. In many cases, your prognosis is actually much better than what the numbers suggest.

Your prognosis does not necessarily determine how *you* will do. It helps you make a treatment decision and understand your situation.

How quickly is my cancer growing?

Doctors estimate how quickly your cancer is growing based on

- the aggressiveness of the cancer cells (the "grade" of the tumor);
- the history of similar cancers (i.e., statistics);
- your personal history (e.g., your lump has doubled in size in one month versus six months).

By looking at your cancer cells under the microscope, doctors can see how closely they look like normal, mature cells. If the cancer cells look mature, they are called "well differentiated." In general, these tend to be slower-growing cancers. If the cancer cells look very immature they are called "undifferentiated" or "poorly differentiated." In general, these are faster-growing cancers. Another term you may hear is "low grade" (slow-growing) or "high grade" (fast-growing).

Well differentiated = low grade (i.e., Grade 1) = slow-growing = indolent
Moderately well differentiated = intermediate-grade (i.e., Grade 2) = moderately fast-growing

Poorly differentiated = high-grade (i.e., Grade 3 or 4) = fast-growing

In addition, the microscopic appearance of the normal cells surrounding the cancer cells sometimes helps to determine the aggressiveness of your cancer. Biochemical, genetic, and immunologic tests are becoming available to better define aggressiveness.

The type of cancer itself may indicate how quickly it is growing or spreading. Certain types of cancer almost always behave aggressively, whereas others usually grow very slowly and rarely metastasize before they are diagnosed and treated. The presence of other medical problems attributed to the cancer (for example, significant weight loss) or certain blood test results may help define the cancer's aggressiveness.

Objective evidence of worsening in a short period of time suggests an aggressive cancer. A cancerous lump that is enlarging quickly, or a spot on a CT or MRI scan that is getting bigger fast, suggests that the cancer cells are multiplying quickly. However, swelling or bleeding around a cancer can cause a lump or spot to enlarge, and may falsely suggest a sudden or significant increase in size of the cancer. A benign (not-cancer) reaction of normal tissue to a small amount of cancer can also make a lump or spot look worse than it is. Further tests usually determine if detectable enlargement is due solely to growing cancer.

Is cancer contagious?

No, cancer is not contagious. You did not catch it from anyone, and it is impossible for you to give your cancer to anyone. If you spend time with children, make this clear right away. Tell your children directly, "Cancer is not catching." Otherwise, they may worry unnecessarily about their own welfare or feel guilty that they caused your illness. Liken cancer to something else that is not contagious such as a broken bone.

What about the types of cancer that are related to viral infections?

Cancer is not infectious, even when it is related to a viral infection. Some types of cancer are related to prior or current viral illnesses because the **virus** changed the genes in a normal cell in a way that predisposed it to becoming cancer years later. In many cases, the patient may have been able to give *the virus* to others during the original infection years ago but the virus has since been cleared from the patient's body. The patient no longer has the virus to give to anyone. The cancer that subsequently develops is not infectious.

In other cases, cancer develops while the viral infection is still present. Hepatocellular carcinoma, a type of liver cancer, occurs more frequently in people chronically infected with the hepatitis B or hepatitis C virus. Certain types of **non-Hodgkin's lymphoma** occur more frequently in people carrying the virus that causes AIDS (HIV). Human papillomavirus (HPV) is associated with cervical cancer. Although the *viruses* associated with these cancers *are* infectious, the cancers that may develop are not communicable. Physicians and nurses who care for cancer patients with AIDS or infectious hepatitis take special precautions to protect themselves from contracting these viruses; they do not need protection from the cancer.

How does cancer start?

Your body is made up of billions of cells that maintain a balance between cell division and cell death. To stay healthy, you are constantly making new hair cells, blood cells, skin cells, and so on. And, by a process called **apoptosis** or programmed cell death, your cells are dying on schedule or when signaled to die by other cells.

Your cancer started in one single cell that developed a *loss of control of cell multiplication and/or cell death*. This single cancer cell made more cancer cells, all of which multiplied too much and died too little. Over time, sometimes months but usually years, the ever-growing population of cancer cells piled up and became big enough to be seen or cause problems. (Note that a cell "multiplies" by "dividing" into two. A loss of control of cell multiplication is the same thing as a loss of control of cell division.)

What causes a normal cell to become a cancer cell?

Cancer is a disease of **genes**, the tiny pieces of DNA (proteins in the chromosomes) in every cell of your body that direct the proper functioning of the cell. Cancer is the result of changes, so-called mutations, in genes that cause these genes to order the cells to divide too quickly and/or not die when they should. Mutations in genes can be inherited (about 20 percent of cancers have a hereditary component) or caused by certain viruses, chemicals, physical agents, or *spontaneous* random genetic events. It is probable that more than one thing has to go wrong to cause a cell to become a cancer cell. Some agents that are associated with the development of cancer don't cause gene mutations but help cancer cells grow.

Once a gene is mutated (changed), is the person destined to develop cancer?

No. Many people inherit mutated genes from their parents, but only some of these people develop cancer. Many people are exposed to known cancer-causing agents, and only some develop cancer. In many cases, this is because most single mutations that are inherited or acquired do not turn a normal cell into a cancer cell all by themselves; the cell must acquire a second or third muta-tion before it becomes cancer. Or, the cell has other features that counteract the ability of the mutation to turn it into a cancer cell.

Can the body repair cancer-causing mutations and prevent a person from developing cancer?

Yes. The body is programmed to repair itself. Your body automat-ically responds to any injury, such as a cut in the skin, with heal-ing processes. Genetic material that gets damaged (such as by UV light or smoking) is usually repaired by the cell before the cell has a chance to become cancer.

Just as some people tend to get thick scars and others heal with barely a trace, people differ in their cells' ability to repair damage to the genes. After a cell becomes cancer, the body's **immune system** often responds by trying to kill the cancer cells before they become numerous enough to become detectable. Some people's immune systems may be more effective at killing or controlling certain cancer cells.

In order to develop detectable cancer, a healthy cell has to have a genetic mutation or combination of mutations that

cause it to become a cancer cell AND the cancer cell has to survive and multiply, without being killed or controlled by your immune system.

What about the role of my environment and lifestyle in causing cancer?

Although the causes of most human cancers remain unidentified, evidence suggests that environmental and lifestyle factors such as smoking, alcohol consumption, and diet contribute to the vast majority. Smoking is, by far, the most powerful link to various cancers. Radiation is responsible for less than 1 percent of cancer deaths, the vast majority of these being attributed to melanoma skin cancer triggered by the sun's ultraviolet rays. Occupational exposure to **carcinogens** (i.e., cancer-causing substances such as asbestos, benzene, or diesel exhaust) in the developed parts of the world has been reduced significantly, now accounting for a very small percentage of total fatal cases of cancer. Some medical treatments such as radiation therapy, chemotherapy, and hormonal therapy may be responsible for about 1 percent of cases of cancer.

Individuals handle cancer-causing agents differently. Exposure to a chemical may cause a lot of genetic damage in one person and little injury in someone else. Many times this is because of differences in how much chemical is converted by the body into harmless substances, and variations in how much chemical is delivered into the cells.

Can I find out what caused my cancer?

We know that some things increase the chance of developing certain cancers:

- The genes you inherited from your parents
- The aging process
- Exposure to carcinogens that damage genes and/or exposure to carcinogens that help cancer cells multiply and spread throughout the body
- Obesity and being overweight; physical inactivity

Cancer is not caused by injuring yourself in ways like bumping your breast, leg, or testicle. An injury may bring a cancer to your attention, but the injury did not cause the cancer.

What are risk factors?

Risk factors increase your chance of developing cancer. A risk factor can be a behavior (such as drinking alcohol or chewing tobacco), an exposure (such as working with certain chemicals or living near a toxic-waste site), an inherited feature (such as fair skin or a family history of colon cancer), or an acquired feature (such as obesity or older age). Most types of cancer have a set of known risk factors for developing that type of cancer. Take note:

- Having a risk factor for your type of cancer does not mean that the risk factor caused your cancer. Many people with known risk factors *never* get cancer, and many people with no known risk factors *do* get cancer.
- Most patients have no risk factors identified for developing their cancer.

What if nobody can explain why I got cancer?

It is natural to look for a cause for your cancer and to search your past for an explanation of what you did wrong. Review with your doctors the list of known risk factors for your type of cancer and address ones that can be modified easily and immediately such as smoking cigarettes or working with carcinogenic substances. Then, from a practical point of view, it is best to focus on getting well again because:

- Finding a cause for your cancer will not affect any of the decisions you make with your doctors about your cancer treatment.
- Finding a cause will not make your cancer go away any faster.
- You cannot change anything that you did in the past.
- Even if you have a known risk factor, there is no way to prove that this is the definite cause of your cancer. Many with this same risk don't develop cancer.
- Blaming yourself doesn't help anyone or anything.

• Time and energy spent looking for a cause is time and energy taken away from adjusting to today and planning for tomorrow.

When faced with a cancer diagnosis, the most helpful question might be: "What can I do about my situation now?"

Am I putting my family at risk for cancer if I do not look for a cause of my cancer?

Some types of cancer have a tendency to run in families. Discuss with your doctor if your family members need to take special precautions or be evaluated in any special way in light of your diagnosis. Some cancers are related to known environmental exposures. Again, ask your doctor if your family needs to evaluate their environment, or undergo any screening tests. These are issues that usually can wait until the flurry surrounding your evaluation has settled down. Do not let a search for a cause for your cancer delay your evaluation and treatment.

Did stress cause my cancer?

Stress does not cause cancer; abnormal genes cause cancer. Most experts (physicians, nurses, social workers, researchers) believe that stress *does* play an important role in your health. But there is no evidence that stress alone causes healthy genes to become cancer-causing genes. When people are diagnosed with cancer after a particularly difficult time in their lives, they may be inclined to blame the strain. Stress *may* have played a role in when the cancer was diagnosed by, for example, affecting your immune system, but the stress did not cause the cancer to develop in the first place. Many people lead extremely stressful lives and never develop cancer.

You cannot change anything in your past. You can only change how you perceive and deal with your world from now on. After you get through this initial phase of adjusting to your illness, you can survey the good and bad stresses in your life. You can determine which distressing situations you can improve or eliminate, and learn how to best manage the unavoidable bad stresses. Dealing with stress in healthy ways may improve your chances for a good response to your cancer therapy. Even if it doesn't, your life will be happier and more comfortable.

Did my diet cause my cancer?

Many foods and diets have been reported to increase the chance of developing cancer. Some foods, dietary habits, and blood levels of vitamins have been shown scientifically to be *associated with* an increased risk of cancer, which just means that they occur together. It is difficult to prove *causation*. For example:

• Alcohol consumption is associated with cancers of the liver, throat, esophagus, mouth, and breast. The risk is increased greatly if the person also smokes.
• High dietary fat is associated with cancers of the colon, rectum, breast, **uterus**, prostate, testes, and gallbladder.
• Nitrites (smoked or salted fish, dried fish, pickled vegetables) are associated with cancers of the stomach and esophagus.
• Salt-cured, smoked, or charred foods are associated with cancer of the esophagus and stomach.
• Low levels in the blood of vitamins A and C are associated with cancers of the esophagus, stomach, colon, rectum, prostate, bladder, lung, and larynx.

Even if your diet is the type associated with an increased risk for your type of cancer, it is still difficult to determine how much your diet contributed to *your* cancer. Many people who follow the same diet don't ever develop cancer. All the information on diet is related to groups of people, not individuals. (For more information about diet and your cancer, see page 117.)

Is my cancer related to AIDS?

People with AIDS (Acquired Immune Deficiency Syndrome) are at increased risk of **Kaposi's sarcoma**, brain lymphoma, high-grade non-Hodgkin's lymphomas, and **invasive** cervical cancer. An HIV or AIDS blood test may be discussed if you have one of these cancers, or if you have risk factors for AIDS, but all these types of cancer also occur in people without AIDS.

Does having cancer put me at increased risk for getting AIDS?

If you are HIV negative and not infected with the virus that causes AIDS, you have the same risk of getting AIDS as you did before your cancer diagnosis. If your cancer therapy requires you to receive blood products, there is an extremely small risk (about 1 in 500,000 units of properly tested units of red blood cells) of transfusion-associated HIV infection, a risk that is outweighed by the risk to your health of not receiving the blood transfusion.

If you are HIV positive, or already have AIDS, your cancer or treatments may suppress your immune system further, thus increasing the risk of AIDS-associated medical problems. All treatment will be aimed at maximizing your chance for survival and maintaining quality of life.

What is the primary lesion?

The place in your body where the first cancer cell arose and then started to grow is called the **primary site**. The cancer that is in the primary site is called the **primary lesion**. Cancers are named after the primary site, even if the cancer cells are found in other parts of the body. For example, cancer cells that started in the colon and then spread (**metastasized**) to the liver are still colon-cancer cells. Sometimes the cancer in the primary site is very small or even undetectable, but doctors know that the cancer started there because of what the cancer cells look like under the microscope or by the results of sophisticated tests done on the cancer cells. Other times when the cancer in the primary site is undetectable, the original site cannot be determined accurately and the patient is said to have a "cancer of unknown primary."

How big is my primary lesion?

The size of the primary lesion is sometimes a factor that helps determine the prognosis, the urgency in treatment, and the options for therapy. If the entire lesion can be removed surgically, its size can be measured directly. If the primary lesion is only biopsied and some of the original cancer is left behind, size is determined indirectly through scans. Sometimes postsurgical changes such as bleeding or swelling can make it difficult to determine the exact size of the cancer on scans.

What if my doctors tell me that they do not know where my cancer started?

Sometimes all the doctors agree about the general type of your cancer (e.g., carcinoma), but they cannot tell where your cancer started (e.g., breast, colon, lung). This is because even with the most sophisticated technology available anywhere in the world, it is impossible to know. In this case, you have a "**cancer of unknown primary**" or "cancer of unknown origin." There are routine procedures for evaluating and treating this situation.

What is the difference between in situ and invasive cancer?

In situ means "in position" and indicates that the cancer is confined and in a very early stage. When viewed microscopically, in situ cancer cells are clumped together, pushing against normal cells but *not invading* local **tissues**. It is not certain that this cancer will ever become invasive and, if it does, the process may take years.

Invasive cancer has spread into healthy tissue, a feature that is determined through microscopic evaluation. Even after certain types of cancer become invasive, they can nevertheless be considered early and curable if still small and **localized** to one small area of the body. As an analogy, a drop of water sitting on top of a sheet of plastic is like an in situ cancer—the water drop is next to the sheet and can be removed completely. A drop of acid sitting on the same sheet of plastic is like an invasive cancer—the acid erodes into the plastic.

What are tumor markers?

Tumor markers are like zip codes for cancer cells, helping to identify their source. Sometimes the presence of a tumor marker or the pattern of tumor markers (i.e., which markers are present and which ones are absent) helps make a specific diagnosis.

When the amount of tumor marker detected in the blood reflects the amount of tumor in the body, it can be used to follow response to treatment. Note: only some types of cancer have tumor markers. Tumor markers can be

- specific proteins on the surface of the cancer cell (e.g., CD antigens);
- specific gene patterns (e.g., BRCA-1 in breast cancer);
- normal cell components released into the blood in abnormal amounts (e.g., LDH).

PSA (prostate specific antigen) is a tumor marker that is used to help screen for and diagnose prostate cancer, follow the response to treatment, and screen for recurrence. Other tumor markers are not specific enough for screening but are very helpful *after* a cancer diagnosis for following the response to treatment and screening for recurrence: e.g., CEA in colon cancer (also elevated in some breast and lung cancers); CA 125 in ovarian cancer; CA 19-9 in pancreatic cancer; beta-2-microglobulin in myeloma and some lymphomas; and alpha-fetoprotein in testicular and liver cancers. Find out if your cancer has any useful tumor markers.

What are lymph nodes?

Lymph nodes are rounded, bean-shaped organs that vary in size from a pinhead to an olive. Thousands of them are scattered throughout your body. As part of your immune system, they help protect you against infection and play a role in your body's immune response to cancer. Many types of cancer can spread to the lymph nodes.

What does it mean if I have lymph node involvement with cancer?

If cancer cells are found in a lymph node, then your cancer has spread beyond the original organ (unless you have lymphoma that started in that lymph node and hasn't spread). Cancer can spread through the blood or lymph to nearby lymph nodes or distant ones. The implications of lymph node involvement may vary depending on many factors, including

- the type of cancer;
- which lymph nodes are involved;
- how many lymph nodes are involved;
- the immune response in the lymph node to the cancer cells.

What does it mean to metastasize? What is a metastasis?

To metastasize is to travel or spread. When cells from the primary (original) cancer break off and spread to another part of the body through the blood or the lymph, they are said to have metastasized. The cancer at the new site is called a **metastasis**. Your physicians may refer to the cancer in the distant organ as a metastasis (plural: metastases). For example, when prostate cancer spreads to the lungs, the spots in the lung are called lung metastases (lung mets for short) and are made up of prostate-cancer cells. Often, metastases in nearby lymph nodes are called positive lymph nodes or lymph node involvement (instead of lymph node mets).

Has my cancer spread (metastasized)?

Tests are done to determine if your cancer has spread (metastasized). If an X ray or scan shows an abnormal spot, it is possible that the cancer has spread to that area. The only way to prove that an abnormality is cancer is to obtain a piece of it with a biopsy, and to examine it. Your doctors can tell you how confident they are that any spots are or are not cancer.

What is a negative test result?

In general terms, a negative test result suggests that you have no abnormalities of what was tested. For example, a chest X ray is called "negative" if there is no evidence of any problems with the lungs, heart, ribs, or lymph tissue in the chest. However, when discussing a test result *with reference to your cancer diagnosis,* "negative" means no evidence of active cancer even if other abnormalities are present. For example, a chest X ray that is negative *for cancer* can show spots of scarred lung tissue, an enlarged heart, or fractured ribs.

negative = normal = not abnormal = not cancer

positive = not normal = abnormal = possibly cancer or definitely cancer (depending on the test)

When told your test results are "negative," make sure you know if they mean negative for any abnormality or just for cancer.

What is a "positive" test result?

A test result is called positive when the test suggests an abnormality of what was tested. In general, the abnormality may be due to cancer or unrelated to your cancer diagnosis. For example, your chest X ray is positive if it shows evidence of viral pneumonia, lung cancer, or a few cracked ribs from falling down the stairs.

However, when discussing a test result (other than a biopsy) *with reference to your cancer diagnosis*, positive means there is an abnormality that *may* be cancer or *is* cancer. If your chest X ray has a new spot in the lung that may be cancer, it is called positive. If a subsequent biopsy shows the spot is malignant (cancer), your chest X ray continues to be called positive. If further tests prove that this spot is benign (not cancer), your chest X ray now is called "negative for cancer" even though it still has an abnormal spot on it. Patients are usually informed of positive results, whether cancer related or not. Note that when discussing the results of a *biopsy* with reference to your cancer, positive always means there is evidence of cancer.

If my scans are negative or normal, does this guarantee that my cancer has not spread to the areas seen on the scan?

No. A negative or normal scan is reassuring but does not guarantee that you are cancer-free in that area. If a cancer is too small, it cannot be detected by these tests. For example, a CAT scan (also called a CT scan) of the liver can pick up spots that are one-half centimeter (approximately one-quarter inch) or bigger in diameter. A normal CAT scan tells you that it is unlikely that there are any areas of cancer one-half centimeter or bigger. Nevertheless, there may be spots of cancer smaller than one-half centimeter in that area. It takes one billion cancer cells to make a lesion one centimeter in size.

After I have a diagnosis, what is the next step?

After you have been diagnosed with cancer through a biopsy or surgery, your doctors may need to perform additional tests to

- determine what stage your cancer is in (see next three questions);
- evaluate for any changes or problems caused by your cancer;
- evaluate your general medical condition unrelated to the cancer.

What is staging?

Staging is the evaluation to determine

- how big your cancer is and how aggressive it is;
- if and to where your cancer has spread.

How is staging done?

Staging is done by

- talking to you (taking a history) and inquiring about specific symptoms;
- doing a physical exam;
- doing various tests and studies (e.g., blood tests, X rays, scans) on you;
- doing various tests on the cancerous tissue that was removed in a biopsy;
- performing additional biopsies or surgery, if necessary.

What does the number of the stage mean?

The higher the stage, the more advanced the cancer. A stage is meaningful only when interpreted for your specific type of cancer.

The implications of stage 3 for your type of cancer may be very different than for stage 3 of another type of cancer. Each type of cancer has its own criteria for determining the cancer stage. Some types of cancer even have a few different staging systems.

Why is staging important?

Cancers of the same type and in the same stage tend to follow the same course. Knowing the stage of your cancer helps your doctors

- know your treatment options;
- determine the best treatment plan for you;
- minimize complications;
- estimate your prognosis;
- communicate with other physicians about your case;
- evaluate your response to therapy;
- contribute to the continuing investigation of cancer.

As advances are being made in our understanding of **oncology**, an increasingly important role in the staging process is being played by the determination of receptor expression, biochemical and genetic markers, hormone status, and immune response to cancer cells. Keep in mind that many factors other than cancer type, grade (how aggressive the cancer cells are), and stage (how far the cancer has spread) determine how you will do.

Are there options regarding the tests used for my staging?

Sometimes. For example, one doctor may suggest noninvasive scans while another recommends surgery to get similar information, or one doctor may want a PET scan instead of a CT scan. Discuss the pros and cons of each option with your doctors. If each strategy seems equally reasonable for assessing your cancer, then other factors will come into play such as scheduling issues, physician preference, and expense.

Do I really need to have all these tests for staging?

You benefit when your doctors know as much as possible about your individual cancer, your overall medical condition, and stage of your disease because:

- Most treatment options are based on the stage of your cancer *and* your medical condition.
- General predictions about your cancer can be made based on the stage of your cancer.
- Potential problems or complications may be discovered; knowing them may allow you to take steps to minimize or avoid them.
- Doctors follow the response of your cancer to any treatments by rechecking these same tests after treatment. For example, if you have a spot on your X ray or scan now and the spot disappears after treatment, then your doctors usually can conclude that the cancer disappeared at that spot.

Incomplete or inadequate staging can lead to "understaging" your cancer and drawing the wrong conclusions about your situation and how best to treat you.

How quickly does my staging need to be done?

The sooner you complete the staging process, the sooner you can talk about your treatment options, make a decision, and begin treatment. Being staged does *not* obligate you to begin treatment. Your staging just provides information that helps you understand your situation and know how quickly you need to make a treatment decision.

Timely, thorough staging is important because:

- Treatment is based on staging, and you usually can't start treatment until you complete your staging. For many cancers, the earlier you start treatment, the better your chance for success.
- Some staging procedures (e.g., surgery) will cause a delay in treatment, so the longer you delay your staging, the longer you are delaying the treatment of your cancer.
- If you begin treatment before your staging is complete, you may lose a marker that could have been helpful in caring for you. Imagine that, after a round or two of treatment, your doctor orders an X ray that you've never had before and it shows a spot. You won't know if the spot is new (i.e., you are not

responding to therapy), or smaller (i.e., you are responding), or unchanged (i.e., your cancer isn't growing but you may need a change in therapy to make it shrink).

How quickly do I need to start treatment?

Your medical condition may necessitate a speedy evaluation so that you can get started on treatment as soon as possible. More often than not, you have *some* time to learn about your cancer and assemble your support group of friends and family before you start treatment. Always keep in mind that while you are not being treated, your cancer is continuing to grow.

How can I get through all these tests while trying to take care of everything else going on in my life?

It's almost impossible to keep up with everything else in your life the same as you did before your diagnosis. In most situations, you shouldn't even try. This is a crisis, even if you feel well and your prognosis is good. Suddenly, your health must take priority over everything else. Although some people can continue their usual home and work responsibilities, most people need to let some things go so that they can give their health the attention it deserves. During a crisis, like any emergency, the rules change regarding who and what get your energy and attention.

Recognize that the immediate situation is temporary even when every day feels like forever. If you take a few days off from work, get behind in your housework, or skip clubs and meetings, it does *not* mean that your life will always be this way. After your evaluation is complete, you will then focus on making a wise decision about treatment. Once you've made a decision with your physicians and your treatment has begun, you can begin a new routine that will once again address all the things that normally go on in your life.

Right now, your top priority is maximizing your chance of getting well and staying well. If you can handle all the testing while keeping up with your usual jobs and responsibilities, great. If you can't do it all, your medical evaluation takes precedence. Later, after you have started treatment, you can manage the fallout of the things you let slip during your evaluation. If you can't decide what things can wait and what needs ongoing attention, ask friends, family, or professionals to help you decide. The next chapter will help you make the best treatment decisions.

2

Making the Best Treatment Decisions

Once your cancer situation has been explained, now what do you do? Before you can begin treatment, you have to figure out what is the best treatment for you. For many people, the time period between making the diagnosis and beginning treatment is the most stressful of all. This is partly because you know that cancer is growing in your body, and you may feel like you aren't doing anything to get better while you are researching your treatment options. Actually, the most powerful steps you can take toward getting better are to become informed about your treatment options, and to invest the time and effort needed to make wise treatment decisions with your doctors. When you make *informed* decisions, you'll never look back saying, "I wish I knew then what I know now!"

Taking time to evaluate your options is best *only if you have the time*; otherwise you may lose your window of opportunity for cure or improvement. If your medical situation warrants immediate treatment, you maximize your chance of recovery by trusting your doctors and beginning treatment now, even if you haven't had time to learn enough to participate in the decisions in any meaningful way.

In this chapter, terms used to describe the goals of treatment, such as **remission** or **cure**, will be defined before reviewing the various treatment options. You will be introduced to methods of making wise treatment decisions including Harpham's Decision Tool for choosing a course of cancer treatment. This grid will help you organize your treatment options in a manageable format, and help you weigh the advantages and disadvantages *to you* of each option. By the end of the chapter, you will have a sense of how to arrive at the best decision *for you* so that you can move into your treatment phase with confidence.

GOALS OF TREATMENT

Why do we treat cancer?

The four reasons to treat cancer are:

• To relieve pain or other symptoms
• To prevent complications from the cancer
• To prevent or slow progression of the cancer
• To cure the cancer

What is a complete remission (CR)?

Also called a complete response, a complete remission is when there is no detectable sign of your cancer. Many people use the term "remission" synonymously with the more accurate phrase "complete remission." All evidence of your cancer may be gone at the end of treatment, during the course of your treatments, or even after diagnostic surgery, such as removal of a tumor in your colon, breast, or lung. Remission is not the same as cure. Many patients achieve a complete remission only to have the same cancer show up again months or years later. Before you are considered cured, you must achieve a complete remission and maintain the remission for a specified amount of time for your particular type of cancer.

What is a partial remission (PR)?

A partial remission is when you still have signs of cancer but your cancer has responded to treatment by shrinking at least in half, with no new areas of cancer and no previous area showing progression. Some people may use the terms "partial remission" or "response" when there is *any* shrinkage of your cancer. Clarify with your doctors what they mean if they use these terms.

What is a minimal remission (MR)?

A minimal remission is the same as a partial remission except your cancer has responded by less than 50 percent.

What is a durable remission?

A durable remission is a complete remission that lasts for a long time. How long "long" is depends on the usual expectations for your type of cancer and is a subjective notion. A durable remission is not the same as a cure. For example, you would be considered to have a durable remission if your type of cancer usually recurs within five years of achieving remission and you've been in remission for eight years. If your type of cancer usually recurs within one year, a three-year remission would represent a durable remission.

What is a molecular remission?

For some types of cancer, sophisticated tests are available in research settings that detect the presence of *even a few cancer cells* in the patient's body. A molecular remission is a remission in which these tests, such as PCR (polymerase chain reaction), do not detect any cancer cells in your body. In contrast, the smallest tumor (i.e., five to ten millimeters) that can be detected by scans contains *billions* of cells.

What is a spontaneous remission?

A spontaneous remission is when cancer disappears by itself without any treatment. This is an unexplained phenomenon that can occur with all types of cancer, more often for some types of cancer compared to others. In all circumstances, remission without treatment is an extremely rare event.

On the one hand, the possibility of spontaneous remission or temporary improvement is one reason why you still can have hope even if no known effective treatments are available for your cancer. On the other hand, to put your hope for recovery in a spontaneous remission instead of available effective therapy would be like hoping to earn money by winning the state lottery instead of getting a job!

What is a cure?

You are considered cured when there is no detectable sign of your cancer *and* you have no more chance of the cancer coming back than if you never had cancer. For some types of cancer, you can be called "cured" if your remission lasts one year. For many other types, five years is the reliable interval after which your chance of recurrence is extremely low. Still other cancers, such as certain types of lymphoma, are considered incurable with current therapies. This is because no matter how long the patient is in remission, the chance of developing the same type of cancer is greater than if the person never had the cancer. Every type of cancer is different. Find out what your doctors mean when they talk about curing your type of cancer.

Is my situation hopeless if my doctors say that my type of cancer is incurable?

No. As long as there is research, your type of cancer is not incurable; it is one of those for which scientists are still working toward a cure. Even if today's treatments for your type of cancer are known to be effective but not curative, available treatments may keep you alive and well while research produces new treatments that *can* cure your disease in your lifetime. Even if curative therapies are not discovered soon, available effective treatments may allow you to live a relatively normal life for a long time, much like people with a chronic disease such as diabetes or heart disease.

As long as there is research, there are no incurable cancers, only those for which scientists are still searching for cures.

What is a recurrence?

You are said to have a **recurrence** if you have been treated for cancer in the past with complete disappearance of all evidence of cancer (you were in complete remission), and now there is evidence that the same cancer has come back. This means that during the time you were in remission you had some remaining cancer cells that were too few or too hidden to be detected at your checkups.

STANDARD AND INVESTIGATIONAL TREATMENTS

How is cancer treated?

Conventional and most investigational treatments involve:

- Surgery
- Radiation
- Medicines
  - • Chemotherapy
  - • Hormonal Agents
    - • supplementing and blocking therapies (for breast and prostate cancer)
    - • cortisone-type steroids
  - • **Biologic therapy** (immunotherapy such as monoclonal antibodies, interferons)
  - • Miscellaneous
- Some combination of the above

What determines which treatments are options for me?

The specific treatment options for your cancer depend on

- your exact diagnosis;
- the stage of your cancer;
- your general medical health, other than your cancer.

What is radiation therapy?

(Radioimmunotherapy is different and will be discussed elsewhere.)

Radiation therapy, also called radiotherapy or irradiation therapy, is based on the ability of X rays (in much higher doses than a standard X ray or CT scan), gamma rays, or electrons to kill cancer cells by damaging their DNA. Radiation is used to cure some cancers, and to control pain in other cancers. It is also used to shrink cancers before surgery, or to mop up any leftover cancer cells in an area after surgery.

Radiation is a local treatment, affecting only the cells in the area of the body that is radiated (the radiation field). The technology of administering radiation therapy continues to improve dramatically. Compared to years ago, many cancers are treated effectively with smaller amounts and more accurate aiming of radiation. This means that patients experience less damage to normal tissue and therefore fewer side effects and late effects (see page 52) than in the past.

What are the different types of radiation therapy?

- External radiation—using a machine outside your body to aim high-energy beams of radiation at spots known to be cancer
- Internal radiation—giving a radioactive source by injection or orally
- Interstitial radiation (brachytherapy)—placing "seeds" of radiation in or near a cancer, either temporarily or permanently

What are the advantages of radiation therapy?

Radiation

- spares most of the normal cells outside the field of treatment the injurious effects of radiation;
- can reach areas that cannot be reached with surgery;
- usually requires a shorter course of therapy than chemotherapy;
- may be an option in people whose medical conditions rule out surgery or chemotherapy as treatment possibilities;
- causes fewer physical changes than with some types of surgery (e.g., mastectomy) or chemotherapy (e.g., hair loss).

What are the disadvantages of radiation therapy?

Radiation

- does not kill cancer cells outside the treatment field;
- usually requires a greater time investment than surgery;

- is available only at hospitals and cancer-treatment centers;
- can cause damage to normal cells in the radiated field, which leads to late effects (see page 53).

What is chemotherapy (chemo)?

Chemotherapy usually refers to medicines that kill rapidly dividing cells such as cancer cells by interfering with their DNA (or RNA or proteins). Chemotherapy can be given by mouth (oral, such as pills and liquids) or by injection into a vein (**intravenous**) or muscle (**intramuscular**). Occasionally, the medicines are injected directly into spinal fluid (intrathecal), into an artery (intra-arterial), or into another part of the body.

What are the main advantages and disadvantages of chemotherapy?

Chemotherapy is systemic, which means that it treats the entire body. When there is reason to believe that you may have cancer cells that cannot be reached with surgery or radiation, chemotherapy has the advantage of giving you the best chance of killing cancer cells anywhere in your body, although some chemotherapy can't get to the brain. The big disadvantage is that chemotherapy is not specific; it works against normal cells that are dividing rapidly, too.

What if the idea of chemotherapy is scary to me?

Technically speaking, chemotherapy is the use of chemicals to treat a disease, so all chemical medicines such as **antibiotics**, blood pressure medicines, and pain medicines are chemotherapy. It may help you to think of chemotherapy as medicine to treat your cancer just as antibiotics treat infection. Some chemotherapy is rough. Other chemotherapy regimens are very mild and well tolerated.

What is hormone therapy?

Hormonal agents are drugs that either supplement (increase) or block (decrease) the effect of certain **hormones** on cancer cells. Some people consider hormone therapy a type of chemotherapy.

Estrogens (female hormone), antiestrogens, androgens (male hormone), antiandrogens, and adrenal inhibitors are used in the treatment of breast and prostate cancer. Adrenocorticosteroids (steroids such as prednisone and dexamethasone) are used as anticancer drugs for a variety of cancers in some chemotherapy regimens. These cortisone-type hormone therapies also are used to help treat a number of cancer-related problems including brain swelling, airway blockage by tumor, vomiting, and poor appetite.

Can I get both chemotherapy and radiation therapy?

Both chemotherapy and radiation, so-called **combined modality therapy**, may be recommended. In order to balance the advantage of improved effectiveness while minimizing the disadvantage of increased toxicity, dosages may be adjusted such as by lowering them and/or spreading them out over a longer period of time. Some situations call for simultaneous chemotherapy and radiation; in other cases, a better outcome is more likely when treatments are administered serially (for example, a course of radiation followed by a course of chemotherapy).

What is biologic therapy (immunotherapy)?

Biologic, or biological, or **immunotherapy**, therapy is a newer approach to treating cancer that is becoming part of standard regimens for some types of cancer but remains purely investigational for other types. It involves giving medicines that boost your own immune system or assist your immune system in killing cancer cells. Biologic therapies include:

- **Interferons** (proteins important in immune function and control of cancer cells)
- **Interleukins** (different proteins that also play a major role in immune function)
- **Monoclonal antibodies**, with or without radioactive or toxic substances attached
- Vaccine therapies (purely investigational)
- **Gene therapies** (purely investigational)

What are monoclonal antibodies?

Monoclonal antibodies are proteins developed in a lab that attach to targets on cancer cells. They are being used to

- help image tumors;
- help purge cancer cells from bone marrow intended for transplant;
- treat specific cancers.

In 1997, the first monoclonal antibody therapy was approved as a cancer treatment (Rituxan® for lymphoma). The advantage of monoclonal antibodies is that they are *relatively* specific for a cell type and relatively nontoxic to cells not of that type. This specificity also means that they work only for the type of cancer for which they were developed. Monoclonal antibodies can be used

- alone ("native" monoclonal antibodies such as Rituxan®, Herceptin®, CamPath®);
- linked to radioactive substances (radioimmunotherapy such as Zevalin® and Bexxar®);
- linked to chemotherapy drugs (antibody-targeted chemotherapy such as Mylotarg®);
- linked to toxins (immunotoxins, in research development).

Studies are under way to determine the best way to use FDA-approved monoclonal antibodies alone and in combination with other standard therapies to control and cure cancer.

What is radioimmunotherapy (RIT)?

Radioimmunotherapy uses radioactive molecules linked to monoclonal antibodies to kill cancer cells. When introduced into a patient's blood, the monoclonal antibodies home in on specific cells, including the cancer cells. Then, the radioactive molecules attached to the antibodies damage the targeted cells. In essence, RIT is a form of systemic radiation therapy. In 2002, Zevalin® became the first radioimmunotherapy to receive FDA approval for the treatment of certain types of lymphoma. Bexxar®, another RIT for lymphoma, is awaiting final FDA approval at the time of this writing.

What is a bone marrow transplant (BMT)?

A **bone marrow transplant**, was the first technique that allowed patients to receive extremely high doses of anticancer therapies. Intense chemotherapy and/or radiation therapy gives patients with some types of cancer (primarily blood cancers) a better chance of obtaining more lasting remissions or cures. These high-dose treatments also destroy the patient's normal bone marrow (the spongy tissue in the middle of bones where blood cells are made). Replenishing the empty marrow with transplanted blood-forming **stem cells** from a donor's marrow is essential to sustain life. A bone marrow transplant is also called a bone marrow rescue or stem-cell transplant, although nowadays the term "stem-cell transplant" usually refers to a peripheral stem-cell transplant (see page 38).

How is a bone marrow transplant done?

First, stem cells are obtained from the marrow in a donor's hip bone (see next question). While the stem cells are being prepared in the lab for transplant into the patient, the patient is given high-dose chemotherapy and/or radiation with the intent of destroying all the cancer cells in the body, wherever they may be. This treatment destroys the normal blood cells in the patient's bone marrow as well as the cancer cells. Then, healthy donor marrow cells are dripped into a vein in the arm like a blood transfusion. The transplanted stem cells circulate in the blood until they set up home in the empty bone marrow and make new, healthy blood.

What is a bone marrow harvest?

This is a surgical procedure done under anesthesia that removes one to two quarts of bone marrow and blood (about 2 percent of the body's marrow) from the bones in the pelvis. The bone marrow can then be used in the next few days, or frozen to be used at a later date.

What is a stem-cell transplant (SCT)?

Also called a peripheral stem-cell transplant (PSCT), a **stem-cell transplant** is a technique that, like the older bone marrow transplant technique, allows the administration of higher doses of anticancer therapies. The advent of growth-stimulating factors has made it possible to collect stem cells from blood drawn from a vein in the arm by a process called **apheresis**. Not only is apharesis less invasive than a bone marrow harvest, but these stem cells also appear to engraft more quickly after being transplanted, thus shortening the hospital stay if all else goes smoothly. Stem-cell transplants now are being done far more often than bone marrow transplants.

What is the difference between autologous and allogenic transplants?

If the stem cells are obtained from the cancer patient (when the patient is in remission) and given back to the patient after he or she receives additional cancer treatment, it is called an **autograft** or **autologous transplant**.

In contrast, if the stem cells are obtained from a healthy donor such as a sibling or an unrelated person, it is called an **allograft** or **allogenic transplant**. Since such a donor's stem cells are not exactly the same as the patient's (unless they are identical twins), the cancer patient's immune system may attack the marrow and cause medical problems, or even reject the new marrow. Another complication of allogeneic transplants may be **graft-versus-host disease (GVHD)**, whereby the healthy donor's marrow cells attack the patient's organs causing mild to life-threatening illness. This graft-versus-host reaction by the donor's healthy marrow is not all bad; it may have some anticancer effect by attacking any leftover cancer cells in the patient's body. A controlled graft-versus-host reaction may confer survival benefits in some cases.

What is a minitransplant or reduced-intensity transplant?

A minitransplant is a type of allogeneic transplant done only in research settings. The patient receives lower dosages of radiation and/or chemotherapy before receiving the stem cells, hence the name "reduced-intensity transplant." Also called nonmyeloablative transplant, transplant-lite, and mixed chimera (half donor, half recipient) transplants, the advantage is that the anticancer treatments given before the transplant are less toxic than those used before standard bone or stem cell transplants. Unlike a standard transplant, which is lethal unless tranplanted stem cells are infused to rescue the marrow, a minitransplant does not destroy the marrow. Donor stem cells are given to attack the remaining cancer cells and not to rescue the bone marrow. Studies are under way to see when minitransplants are the best option for a patient.

What are umbilical cord transplants?

Investigational studies suggest that newborns' blood obtained from the umbilical cord may provide a source of healthy blood-making cells for bone marrow damaged by high-dose cancer treatments. These stem cells are available at no risk to the infant donor and are far less likely to contain infectious agents than stem cells obtained from an adult's marrow. Scientists are researching ways to overcome the limits imposed by the small amount of blood available from each umbilical cord. Studies are looking at whether newborn stem cells are hardier and more effective factories of healthy blood cells over the long term than adult stem cells.

What is targeted therapy?

The ideal cancer therapy is targeted therapy: treatment that kills only cancer cells and spares healthy cells. Targeted therapies cause fewer side effects, complications, and late effects. Research is investigating targeted medicines that will

- attach to or interact with substances that are present *only* in cancer cells;
- interfere with processes that occur *only* in cancer cells and are necessary for cancer cells to divide or survive.

Gleevec®, a drug that blocks an enzyme needed by chronic myeloid leukemia (CML) cancer cells, was the first targeted therapy to receive FDA approval and became available in 2001. Iressa, a targeted therapy for lung cancer, is nearing release.

What are cancer vaccines?

Although these vaccines are not yet available as standard treatment, research studies are under way to develop ones that can treat active cancer or prevent recurrent cancer. Cancer vaccines use small amounts of cancer cells, part(s) of cancer cells, or product(s) of them to stimulate your immune system to recognize and kill cancer cells in much the same way that the polio vaccine uses polio proteins to stimulate your immune system against the polio virus. One of the major benefits will be that vaccines, if effective, can have long-lasting effects. Some vaccines will be mass-produced to work against a type of cancer in many different patients; other vaccines will be custom-made from an individual's tumor and will work only for that individual patient.

What is gene therapy?

Gene therapy is another promising treatment being studied in research settings. The goal of gene therapy is to change the genetic makeup of cancer cells so that the cancer cells (and not the normal cells)

- are more susceptible to anticancer therapies;
- cannot multiply;
- cannot spread to other parts of the body;
- die without any further therapy.

Other gene therapies may be used to change the genetic makeup of the normal cells (and not the cancer cells) so that the

- normal cells are protected from the damaging effects of anticancer therapies;
- immune system is more efficient at killing cancer cells.

One particularly promising area of gene research is "antisense therapy" in which proteins are given in hopes of blocking the ability of oncogenes (cancer genes) to signal the cell to become cancerous.

What are angiogenesis inhibitors (antiangiogenesis agents)?

Tumors depend on a blood supply to grow and spread. Angiogenesis inhibitors are being developed in research laboratories to take advantage of the differences between normal blood vessels and those that grow into and around tumors. Blocking the growth of a tumor's blood vessels should starve the tumor to death and leave normal tissue unscathed. Even if angiogenesis inhibitors can't get rid of the cancer, it is hoped that they will be able to prevent tumors from growing or spreading to other parts of the body. As long as your cancer is not interfering with vital structures and functions, you can live a relatively long and normal life.

What if my oncologist says that these newer therapies aren't available to me?

When you hear about promising new treatments that are still in the research stage of development, remember that they have not yet been proven to be at least as safe and effective as current therapies. Their *potential* benefits over current therapies make them newsworthy. They nourish the real hope that better therapies will be available to you and your loved ones in the future. You may want to find out about **clinical trials** (see page 44).

Are my treatment options standard?

A treatment option is *standard* when it is recommended routinely. Each standard cancer therapy is the result of years of well-controlled studies, and is *proven* to be relatively safe and effective. Doctors can provide information on the risks, side effects, and chances of success for each standard therapy. Advantages of standard therapy include:

- It may give you the best chance of cure or improvement.
- Doctors have more experience with it, so they can prepare you for what is involved.

- It is available at most facilities that treat cancer patients.
- It is usually covered by insurance.

Other terms used for **standard** therapy are **conventional** and "mainstream" therapy. The terminology gets tricky. When conventional therapies such as radiation and chemotherapy are used in unconventional ways, they are no longer considered standard therapy.

Does it matter where I receive standard treatment?

Any location is only as good as the treatment available and the doctors working there. You must consider the doctor's expertise in the type of cancer that you have.

Your treatment may last many months to years. The closer to home that you can receive treatments, the easier it will be for you and your family. Some people start their treatments in a large medical center far from home, and then continue their treatments in a smaller local medical facility. Some treatments are available only at certain hospitals or centers.

How true are all the unpleasant stories about conventional therapies?

Advances in cancer therapy include great strides in preventing and treating the side effects of therapy. Pain initiatives have encouraged professionals to be proactive in the use of available methods of effective pain control. Excellent antinausea medicines are available now that were not available in the early 1990s. The increasing attention focused on nutrition and exercise in cancer survivors undergoing treatment has led to a better understanding of effective methods to help keep your body well nourished and conditioned. Support groups and self-help books can help you to understand and deal with the psychosocial issues of undergoing cancer treatment.

If you hear unpleasant stories, remember that people treated before 1990 did not have access to the same medicines to deal with side effects as are currently available. If a person received different treatment or had a different type of cancer, you can expect a different experience. Even if everything about another person is similar (same age and sex patient, same type of cancer, same stage of cancer, same therapy, same general health), you are still a different person. Your response to your therapy is unique.

As is true of most other life experiences, your attitude and expectations can make a difference. If you go into chemotherapy expecting to be very sick, you probably will be. If you go into it with optimism, you may have a better chance of milder symptoms.

Conventional therapies have made it possible for millions of cancer survivors to enjoy healthy lives today.

What is investigational treatment?

When a drug or a treatment is under study, it is called investigational or **experimental**. Oncologists around the world are conducting studies on patients using:

- New combinations of old drugs or treatments
- New ways of administering old drugs (such as with higher doses, constant **infusions**, or infusions directly into a tumor)
- Completely new drugs or treatments
- New drugs or treatments in combination with old drugs or treatments

Investigational therapy is *not* the same as unconventional therapy, alternative therapy, or complementary therapy (see pages 72 and 80).

What is informed consent?

Informed consent is your competent and voluntary written approval to receive treatment *after* you have received information that allows you to understand

- the nature of the treatment;
- the purpose of the treatment;
- the benefits, short-term and long-term;
- the risks, short-term and long-term;
- the expense, short-term and long-term;
- the other options available to you.

What are clinical trials of cancer therapies?

After investigation has shown a drug or treatment to have some antitumor effect in lab (test-tube or animal) tests, the promising new treatment is studied in trials involving human patients. These investigational studies, called clinical trials, are aimed at finding safer and more effective treatments for all the different types of cancer, and are administered by highly trained, highly qualified doctors. With time, treatments that prove to be safer or more effective become the new standard treatment.

Can I be treated in a clinical trial without my knowing it?

No. All participants must give written informed consent before beginning any treatments.

Why would I want to enter a clinical trial?

If your type of cancer is not reliably or easily cured with standard therapy, clinical trials may offer you unique advantages, such as:

- Possibly receiving a treatment that subsequently proves to give you the best chance for doing well
- Providing an opportunity to try newer treatments before they are generally available
- Offering a chance to participate in work that helps all cancer survivors, no matter the medical outcome for individual participants or the conclusions drawn from the trial
- Financial relief when the trial being considered provides all treatment and follow-up at no cost to the patient (not all trials do this, and some trials become financially prohibitive for many people when travel costs are involved)

What is the difference between phase-I, -II, and -III trials?

The earliest trials, phase-I trials, are designed *to determine the safety* of a new treatment, not its effectiveness against cancer. These trials are generally reserved for a few people with very advanced cancers who have little hope of relief or cure with standard therapy. After a medication or treatment has been shown to be safe in a phase-I trial, it can be given in phase-II trials. These trials involve larger numbers of people and are designed to *determine whether these treatments have any effectiveness* against specific types of cancer. When a treatment has been shown to be safe and demonstrates some effectiveness, it enters phase III. Phase-III trials are designed *to determine if a new treatment is better* than standard therapy.

Should I consider investigational treatment for my cancer?

You should consider investigational treatment if

- you have a rare cancer;
- your chances for cure or remission are low with standard therapy; or
- you live near a cancer center that is conducting clinical trials.

When should I consider the option of entering a phase-I trial? Phase II? Phase III?

Phase-I and -II trials should be considered only if there are no effective standard therapies available to you. Simply put, the benefits of standard therapies are proven and measurable; the benefits of investigational treatments in phase-I and -II trials are completely unknown. If a standard treatment is available for your cancer that offers you a high likelihood of cure or some good quality time (months or years), this treatment is usually a better choice than entering a phase-I or -II trial. Standard therapy usually delays disability and death due to cancer. Not only do you have this time to live, but you also increase your chance of being around to benefit from more effective therapies that become available to you in phase-III trials, or as new standard therapy in the future.

Unlike phase-I and -II, phase-III trials usually can offer *at least* as much benefit as standard therapy in the prevention or treatment of cancer and its complications. Consider looking into available phase-III trials for your type of cancer if standard therapies

- rarely result in cures;
- rarely result in durable (long-lasting) remissions;

- are extremely toxic; or
- are often associated with serious late effects (see page 52).

Are people who participate in clinical trials "guinea pigs"?

No. You cannot become a participant in a clinical trial without your written informed consent, let alone without your knowledge. You would *never* be given a placebo (i.e., an inactive substance) instead of known effective anticancer treatments. If unexpected problems arise with your condition, or with other patients in the trial, the trial may be stopped prematurely. When you participate in a trial, *your personal safety is of paramount importance* even though trials are designed to discover basic truths about treating cancer.

Once I participate in a clinical trial, am I obligated to stay in the trial?

No. Participation in a clinical trial is voluntary. You can drop out of a study at any time without jeopardizing your medical care. You have every right to do what is best for you, physically, emotionally, and financially. If, during the study, it becomes obvious that participation is no longer the best treatment for you, you will be removed from the study, or you can remove yourself. However, agreeing to participate in a clinical trial implies a level of commitment. It takes manpower, equipment, and money to run a clinical trial. When participants drop out, conclusions may be weaker or impossible to draw, and costs are increased.

What about the media reports of improper enrollment or treatment of patients resulting in unnecessary injury and death?

In recent years, a few isolated tragic events in research settings precipitated a dramatic overhaul of the system that protects patients. The grievous errors of a few individuals can't diminish the unique and invaluable benefits of clinical trials. In response to reports of research fraud, oversight committees have been established to perform rigorous audits of all clinical-trial data. New, sophisticated procedures are being employed to ensure high-quality, accurate data collection, monitoring, and auditing.

Who runs clinical trials?

In the United States, clinical trials are overseen by

- the National Cancer Institute, or
- a "cooperative group," an organized group of oncologists from a number of hospitals and clinics, who are trained in designing, running, and interpreting clinical trials, or
- a qualified individual oncologist or group of oncologists in one institution or clinic.

What are the downsides of clinical trials?

There are some potential disadvantages to participating in a clinical trial:

- You may lose an opportunity for a dependable response from standard therapy if you pursue a clinical trial of therapy that proves to be less successful than standard therapy.
- By definition, not all the side effects and risks are known ahead of time.
- There is less predictability of success in phase-I and -II trials; in phase-III studies, success is expected to be at least as good as with standard treatment, but still it is uncertain.
- Doctors have less experience working with investigational and new treatments than with standard, established ones.
- Clinical trials require an investment in terms of your time, energy, and testing to comply with the required follow-up during and after treatment.
- Hospitalization may be required for some treatments.
- Trials can add to emotional stress (for example, if you don't know exactly which treatment you are getting).
- Some people feel like "a number" instead of an individual human being. (Note that other trial participants feel that they get even *more* individualized attention than they would if they received standard treatment.)
- Availability is restricted (trials are available only at certain centers).
- There are possible problems with insurance reimbursement

(although some clinical trials treat patients at no charge) and the nonmedical expenses that aren't covered.
- Physician referral is needed.

Why doesn't everyone who has cancer that is not easily curable with standard therapy participate in clinical trials?

Clinical trials are not for everyone. There are practical reasons why more people do not participate in trials, including:

- Standard conventional treatment may be safer or more effective for them.
- People may be unaware of their availability and benefits.
- Trials have limited participation; ongoing trials may have no openings.
- Many people don't qualify for trials applicable to their type of cancer because of their age or concurrent medical conditions.
- People may choose not to participate because of family constraints, or the financial and emotional burden of being away from home.
- People may choose not to participate because of the stress associated with the added uncertainties of trial treatments.
- Some oncologists discourage their patients from participating.

How can I find out which clinical trials are available?

You and your doctors can find out about available clinical trials related to your cancer by consulting:

- **PDQ** ("Physician Data Query") of the National Cancer Institute, a frequently updated computerized list of ongoing trials. Call toll-free 800-4-CANCER or go to www.cancer.gov/search/clinical_trials/
- OncoLink at www.oncolink.com/templates/treatment/matching.cfm or call 877-601-8601
- The oncology research departments of major cancer centers, and inquiring if they are conducting any trials for your type of cancer that are not registered with the NCI

- Pharmaceutical companies involved in cancer research who may be conducting trials that are not sponsored by the NCI and, therefore, are not listed in PDQ

How do I decide if I want investigational treatment?

Learn about clinical trials for your type of cancer, especially if you don't like any of your standard options. If you are eligible for a trial that looks appealing, compare the risks and benefits of this option *for you* against standard treatments (see page 32 on making a treatment decision). Although trials are not available for all patients, and investigational therapy is not the wisest choice for everyone, patients who never consider this option may be bypassing what would have been their best treatment option.

Most people who consider the possibility of entering a clinical trial (see page 44) ultimately receive standard treatment. Sometimes this is because no trials are open at the time they need to begin treatment or they don't meet the criteria for entering the ongoing trials. For many people, standard therapy is the better option given the specifics of their situation.

Do I have any other options if standard therapy offers me little hope of improvement or cure *and* I am not a candidate for any of the clinical trials that are now accepting patients?

Yes. You may be a candidate for a drug or treatment that your doctor can obtain for you under the FDA's "compassionate use" guidelines. These drugs are very new, and their safety and efficacy are less certain, but they may offer you more hope than standard therapy.

When standard and investigational treatment options in the United States have been exhausted, some people contact one of the private enterprises that, for a fee, will provide a list of trials and treatments available worldwide, outside of the American medical system. This should only be pursued as an option of last resort when in an otherwise hopeless situation. Most oncologists discourage this option.

Before making any treatment decisions, discuss your treatment options with your doctors.

Why are some treatments available only outside the United States?

In addition to standard American medical treatments and treatments involved in clinical trials, cancer treatments are being given outside the American medical mainstream. These treatments are not subject to the same stringent regulation as in the United States. The main reasons for FDA regulation in the United States are to protect you from

- ineffective treatment, especially when effective treatment is available;
- dangerous treatment, especially when less dangerous treatment is available; and
- unscrupulous individuals who want to exploit you for financial gain.

An unintended consequence of strict regulation is that a superior new treatment might become available outside the United States before it is available here.

There are many practical problems inherent in being treated outside the American medical mainstream:

- Difficulty finding an American doctor to administer the treatments
- The need to travel, often far distances, with its great expense, separation from your support system (friends and family), and possible language problems
- Possible problems with insurance reimbursement

MAKING THE TREATMENT DECISION

What do doctors mean when they talk about the risks of treatment?

Cancer treatments can cause a variety of unintended consequences—from minor skin irritation to life-threatening infections. Your doctors may use the word "risk" in a number of different ways. They may mean danger or threat, as in "There is a risk of nerve damage." Your doctors may also use the word "risk" to mean a possible problem, as in "One risk of this particular chemotherapy is nerve damage." When the word is used in this way, you have no indication of how likely nerve damage is or how serious the nerve damage would be. A third way doctors use the word "risk" is when quantifying the possibility of a problem, as in "There is a seventy-five percent risk (chance or likelihood) of developing nerve damage."

Every time a medical decision is made, the potential benefits are weighed against the risks. As new therapies are first used in large numbers of patients, unforeseen risks may become apparent as well as unforseen benefits.

What are the short-term risks of each treatment option?

Each treatment option carries risks of **side effects** and **complications**. Side effects are unfavorable symptoms or changes that *may* commonly arise during treatment, such as nausea, hair loss, sore mouth, and fatigue. Complications are problems that arise, are due to your disease or treatment, and may threaten your health or life. Examples of complications include infection, dehydration, blood clots, and poor healing of incisions.

Your risk of developing specific side effects or complications depends on

- which treatments are used;
- your type of cancer;
- how advanced your cancer is;
- the presence or absence of any other medical conditions, such as heart, lung, or kidney problems;
- medications you are taking for non-cancer-related conditions;
- other factors that are hard to measure.

Remember: Everyone is different. Statistics cannot predict which side effects or problems, if any, you will have with any given course of treatment. Millions of people have gone through cancer treatments and now enjoy healthy lives, including those who experienced side effects or complications.

Will my evaluation or treatment affect my ability to have children, now or later?

Some tests and treatments for cancer affect the ability of a man to produce sperm, or the ability of a woman to get pregnant or have a normal pregnancy. Some diagnostic tests and cancer treatments pose risks to the unborn child conceived or carried at the time. Although fertility may be the farthest thing from your mind right now, you may need to address it so that in the future you do not regret any decisions you make today. You want to be able to look back and know that you made informed decisions.

Note: If there is any chance that you are pregnant, tell your physicians immediately!

Are there any precautions I can take to minimize the risk to my fertility?

Ways to minimize the risk to your fertility include the following:

- When two or more equally good tests or treatments are available, choose the one that carries the least risk regarding fertility.
- Inquire whether any of your tests and treatments involving irradiation can be done with extra shielding.
- If you are a woman about to undergo surgery before radiation to your abdomen, inquire whether your surgeon can tack your ovaries out of the field of intended radiation, and thus decrease exposure of your eggs to radiation.

Can I save ("bank") my sperm or eggs?

If there is concern that future fertility may be impaired, you should discuss saving your sperm or (fertilized) eggs *before* you receive any treatments. You may want to contact a medical center or physician specializing in fertility to get the most up-to-date information.

What are late effects?

Late effects are changes and problems that first appear months or years after completion of cancer therapy, and are due to the cancer or its treatment. Examples of late effects include infertility and premature menopause due to certain types of chemotherapy, scarring due to surgery or radiation, premature heart disease following radiation to the heart, and the most feared late effect of all—a second cancer due to certain types of radiation or chemotherapy.

The idea of late effects can be distressing when trying to decide on a course of cancer treatment. Use facts to help you maintain a healthy perspective:

- Most long-term survivors do *not* develop serious late effects.
- The late effects being seen in today's long-term survivors often are due to treatments that are now obsolete, having been replaced by safer, less toxic therapies such as the ones you might be receiving.
- Research is finding ways to prevent, minimize, detect early, and treat late effects.
- Late effects only occur in people whose lives were saved from cancer. From the perspective of someone with cancer for whom there are no effective treatments, late effects are a luxury reserved for long-term survivors of an otherwise fatal condition.

What causes late effects?

Late effects can develop when normal, healthy cells are killed by treatment aimed at cancer cells, or when healthy cells are injured and cannot repair themselves completely.

If cancer treatment can cause late effects, why don't doctors give lower doses of treatment in order to eliminate the chance of developing late effects?

All cancer treatment seeks to strike the best balance between the cure or control of the original cancer and the prevention of complications from the therapy. Finding the optimal treatment for you is like walking a tightrope: If you receive too little cancer therapy in the hope of sparing you late effects, you increase your chance of dying from treatable or curable cancer because of undertreatment; if you receive too much therapy in the hope of ensuring a cure of your cancer, your risk is increased of dying from the treatment (now or later) or surviving with an unacceptably compromised quality of life. Ideal cancer treatment would kill only cancer cells and leave normal cells unscathed. Researchers are working hard to develop these so-called targeted therapies.

Can I do anything now to help prevent the development of serious late effects?

You may decrease your risk of developing late effects compared to others getting the same treatments by

- obtaining state-of-the-art conventional therapies with state-of-the-art equipment;
- keeping your blood pressure well controlled during and after radiation therapy;
- avoiding cigarettes, excessive alcohol, and other substances known to be injurious to the body;
- taking your medicines exactly as prescribed;
- reporting to your oncologist immediately when you become aware of something that may affect the safety of your treatments (for example, if you are becoming dehydrated, or if you accidentally take too many pills);
- discussing with your physicians any available measures to prevent or screen for late effects once your treatments are completed.

Research scientists are investigating the safety and efficacy of treatments given along with conventional therapies in the hope of preventing late effects. You may want to consider participating in a clinical trial so that you could possibly receive one of these new treatments. A patient-oriented discussion of late effects can be found in my book on recovery and long-term survivorship, *After Cancer: A Guide to Your New Life* (HarperCollins).

Will my age affect my treatment options?

Maybe. Normal, unavoidable age-associated changes in the body increase the risks of some treatments. Upper age limits are set when it is felt that the risks of intensive treatments such as stem-cell transplants may outweigh their potential benefits. As technology and supportive therapies continue to improve, the cutoff age can be expected to increase.

At your age, will aggressive treatment add more quality or quantity of life than less aggressive treatment? For an eighty-five-year-old person with a slow-growing cancer, less aggressive treatment may offer the same (or better) life expectancy and a much better quality of life than intensive treatment would provide. Note that recent studies suggest that elderly patients who are otherwise healthy can tolerate most standard cancer therapies. If you feel that your oncologist is withholding reasonable treatment options because of your age, get a second opinion.

What if I don't want to hurt my body by taking toxic treatment?

It is normal and adaptive to want to avoid damaging your body. If you had never developed cancer, you would never have wanted to expose yourself to surgery, chemotherapy, or radiation. Now that you have cancer, *the equation has changed*: If you don't take effective cancer therapy, you will probably die of your cancer. When standard cancer therapies can help you, they are not toxic poisons but healing medicines.

Cancer treatments are bad for healthy people.
Cancer treatments are good for people with cancer.

What if I get upset even thinking about the possibility of side effects, complications, or late effects?

Talking about the risks of cancer treatment can be frightening and anxiety provoking. That is because the risks are being laid out in front of you, and you have to concentrate on them in order to make a rational treatment decision. Rest assured that once your treatments are started you will probably find it easier to push the possible risks into the background and focus on getting well again. Dealing with your fears and anxieties is discussed more fully in chapter 5. When you have cancer, you have to take some risks in order to get well again.

After you make your treatment decision by weighing all the risks and benefits of your options, you will be able to focus your attention on the benefits of your final choice.

What are second opinions?

Second opinions are evaluations by different doctors who review your case and give you their conclusions about your situation and treatment options. Having someone else examine your medical situation allows you to review all your treatment options, provides an opportunity to draw or confirm your conclusions, and helps you to feel more confident about these important decisions.

Why would I want a second opinion?

You probably rely on additional opinions when you are making other important decisions. For example, you may read *Consumer Reports*, talk with friends, and do some comparative shopping before buying a car. Or, if a mechanic told you that you needed an eight-hundred-dollar part to fix the clank in your car, you might take your car to a second shop for another opinion before agreeing to the repair. Obviously, your health is infinitely more valuable than your car.

Do I need a second (or third, or fourth) opinion?

As long as you are not risking life or limb by delaying treatment for a short while, a second opinion should be obtained if you desire another opinion and/or your insurance company requires one. Deciding what to do about your cancer is such an important decision that many people seek a second opinion even if they have a very common cancer and a good prognosis with standard treatment.

At least one other opinion is strongly recommended if:

- Multiple treatment options are available for you.
- Your prognosis is not good with the proposed treatment.
- The treatment recommended carries significant risk.

- The treatment will affect your lifestyle.
- You feel rushed into a decision.
- You feel the slightest lack of confidence in the doctor or the recommended treatment.

If I decide to get a second opinion, do I have to go through all the tests again?

Usually the second opinion can be based on all the test results obtained during your initial evaluation (biopsy results, scans, and the rest). Sometimes additional studies are requested by the doctors giving the second opinion. Studies you've already had would be repeated only if the first study did not provide adequate information. This can happen because of a problem with artifact (for example, if the angle wasn't perfect or some movement occurred during the scan) or sampling (the biopsy didn't get a big enough piece of the cancer to make a definitive diagnosis). Or, the doctors may be concerned about the possibility of a significant change since the time of the studies, a change that would affect their advice. This may happen if a lot of time has elapsed or you have a fast-growing cancer.

What are the advantages of getting a second opinion?

Each doctor has a unique perspective on your illness because of his or her training and experience. Second opinions may provide:

- Confirmation of the first opinion. This helps you feel more confident, now and later, about the decisions you make.
- Additional information that helps support the first opinion.
- The introduction of an additional option that you (a) decide is best for you or (b) consider and then reject in favor of the treatment recommended originally. Thereafter, if you read or hear about this other option, you will feel comfortable that you considered it and made the best decision for you.
- The opportunity for you to meet another oncologist whom you would prefer to care for you.

What are the downsides to getting a second opinion?

It can be emotionally draining to gather and sort through complex and frightening information needed to make life-and-death decisions. It consumes time and energy. It can be expensive due to travel and time off from work.

The oncologist providing the second opinion may present a more gloomy interpretation of your prognosis and treatment options than your original oncologist. Or the second oncologist's style and philosophies may differ from yours, making the experience unpleasant or upsetting. Even though you may dismiss these opinions as not valuable for you, it may be hard to forget what was said, especially when you're going through some rough spots.

You may feel anxious about your cancer growing while you are getting second opinions. You may feel an urgency to get started on treatment right away. For most people, the cancer has been present for months or years before it was first detected. As long as your medical condition is stable, and your doctors feel that you are not jeopardizing your health by delaying treatment for a few days or weeks, you do have time.

Another common problem is that you may receive conflicting information or advice from second opinions. You are now faced with sorting out which information to believe and which advice to follow. This can be extremely stressful until you make your final decision, especially if you are feeling overwhelmed by the diagnosis or all the new medical terms and procedures. In the long run, your effort will be rewarded with the comfort and confidence that accompanies making thoughtful decisions on the basis of the best information available at the time.

In most cases, the lifelong benefits of making an informed decision far outweigh the short-term disadvantages.

Why might the oncologist providing the second opinion disagree with my original oncologist?

When doctors disagree on how to manage your situation, it's because there is no single best treatment. When treatments are fairly new, definitive answers about long-term risks and benefits are not available. In addition, each doctor's conclusions and advice regarding your situation are based on many factors, including the physician's

- personal clinical experience (the successes and failures seen personally with various treatments);
- personal involvement in clinical research;
- individual interpretation of the available data (different doctors can draw different conclusions from the same data);
- community's standards of care (regional variations exist in how and when specific treatments are used).

How do I decide what to do if the oncologist providing the second opinion disagrees with my original oncologist?

If you get conflicting advice, ask each oncologist to explain his or her advice in light of their differences. You can determine how simple or elaborate an explanation you want or need. After sorting through the various recommendations, hopefully all the physicians will agree that there is one best choice or a few equally good choices.

Unfortunately, sometimes doctors disagree about what is best for you. Even after discussion, one may suggest that his or her advice is best and that the other option is a wrong choice for you. Since everyone cannot be right, you may have to dismiss the advice of one or more of the doctors in order to proceed. Whom do you believe? How do you decide what is the best course of action? Additional second opinions (third and fourth opinions) may resolve the conflict. How you feel (your intuition or gut feeling) may help guide you to the best choice for you.

Since part of the problem may be that you and your oncologist don't know each other well yet, discussing the situation with your longtime internist or family practitioner may be helpful. The confidence and trust that have developed over the years are powerful forces, and the input of a personal physician may be very helpful. Even when, as is often the case, they don't feel qualified to recommend a specific course of treatment, they may be able to help you work through the advantages and disadvantages of your choices, or reassure you about the caliber of your oncologist.

You always have options. The key to making wise choices is discussing your options with well-qualified physicians whom you trust and, together, arriving at a plan of action.

What if my family wants me to pursue a second opinion and I don't feel the need?

There are many reasons, rational and emotional, for you and your family to feel the way you do. Open, honest communication is the key to getting you the best medical care possible and enjoying the support of those who care about you. It might be helpful if you involve an impartial observer such as a social worker or counselor experienced in helping people make medical decisions. The bottom line is that *you* make the final decisions about which doctors you see or which treatments you pursue, if you are well enough to make decisions.

Will my doctors be upset or angry if I seek a second opinion?

You don't have to worry about a doctor's feelings when you request another opinion. Doctors are here to help you. Oncologists expect their patients to get second and third opinions when the patient or the patient's family feels the need. If you sense disapproval on the part of your doctor when you request a second opinion, step back and see whether you are perhaps interpreting your self-consciousness as your doctor's disapproval. If you are sure that your doctor is unhappy about your getting another opinion, consider switching doctors. Unless life or limb is in immediate danger without treatment, it is a red flag when your doctor urges you not to get a second opinion or threatens to stop caring for you if you do. This is an especially difficult situation if you live in a small town with only one or two available oncologists.

If you find yourself going from doctor to doctor, never feeling satisfied with the advice or the care that you receive, get professional counseling to help you learn how to assess your options and make decisions about your care.

Second opinions are part of cancer survivorship. You have a right to be as sure as possible about decisions that affect your life.

Can I obtain a second opinion without telling my oncologist?

Yes, but it's not a good idea. The essence of the doctor-patient relationship is mutual trust. It is best to keep everything aboveboard. There are practical considerations, too: The doctor providing the second opinion will likely need some information that is available only from your oncologist, such as the results of your physical exam when you were first seen. In addition, it could be awkward for you if your oncologist found out that you went for another opinion and tried to keep it a secret.

How do I arrange for a second opinion?

You can be referred to an oncologist for a second opinion by:

- Your current doctors
- Friends who have been treated for cancer
- Your local medical society
- The American Cancer Society
- The National Cancer Institute's Cancer Information Service (CIS) at 800-4-CANCER
- Cancer centers that accept self-referrals by patients

How do I prepare for a second opinion?

You can save time and money, and enhance the value of your second opinion, with some simple preparation. Arrange to have copies of your medical records, pathology slides, scans and their interpretation, and other test results delivered to the consultant so that they can be reviewed *before* your scheduled visit. Check with the consultant's office to make sure your records arrived and to see if there might be anything else he or she needs prior to your visit.

When you go for your second opinion, keep an open mind. See the consultation as a good opportunity to obtain more information about your situation and treatment options as well as to hear a new opinion about what is the best approach for you. Information and advice from experts help you make wise decisions.

How do I decide which treatment option to pursue?

When talking with your physicians, you will develop a good sense of what your best treatment option is by reviewing with your physicians the answers to the following questions:

- What are the treatment options available to me, both conventional and investigational?
- What is the remission rate of each option? How long do remissions usually last?
- What is the response rate of each option (partial and complete remissions)?
- What is the cure rate of each option?
- What are the short-term risks of each option?
   What is my risk of dying?
   What are the potential side effects and complications?
- What are the long-term risks of each option?
   What is my risk of developing a second cancer?
   What is my risk of developing a serious medical problem such as heart, lung, or kidney disease?
   What is my risk of developing a less serious medical problem that would be significant to me (e.g., numbness in the fingertips that would make it difficult for a violinist to perform)?
- What future options are compromised or eliminated by each treatment option? (After certain treatments, other treatments can have a lower success rate, carry greater risk, or are no longer options.)
- Who can provide the treatment?

- Where can I receive treatment?
- How long is each treatment course?
- How debilitated will I be from treatment?
    Will I be able to work?
    Will I be able to pursue my special interests?
- How much will it cost?

The best choice for treatment depends on your desires, values, goals, and personal risk-taking preferences. For some people, the right choice is treatment with a goal of cure no matter what the chance for cure (as long as there is some chance) and no matter what the risks and costs of treatment. For others, going for the cure is not the best route because the chance for cure is very low, and the price (discomfort, travel, expense, risk of death or complications) is too great. You may decide that your best choice at this time is taking a treatment that *controls* your cancer without curing it, especially if this treatment doesn't eliminate other options should it stop working.

Doctors can provide some statistical data for each treatment option regarding your chances of remission, cure, complications, side effects, and death. Doctors and nurses can give you some concept of what the experience of treatment will be like. Patients who have been through similar treatments can give you a closer insight into the experience. Your doctors or nurses usually can refer you to patients willing to share with you their experiences and advice. Be sure to ask for the names of patients who have completed their treatment as well as patients currently under treatment.

If you were basically healthy before your diagnosis of cancer, the key question is: *Which treatment will give you the greatest chance of cure or longer life, and at what price?*

What if I'm finding it hard to balance the advantages and disadvantages of my treatment options to decide on the best course?

All the information about remission rates, side effects, complications, risks, and so on can be overwhelming. I designed Harpham's Decision Tool to help patients make treatment decisions. It is a simple grid that enables you to compare all the key information on one page. Harpham's Decision Tool helps when you have more than one treatment option, none of which is clearly the best. You may find it especially helpful when you don't like *any* of your options.

In the grid below, fill in each box with a rating:

+ + + + = very big advantage	- - - - = very big disadvantage
+ + + = big advantage	- - - = big disadvantage
+ + = advantage	- - = disadvantage
+ = slight advantage	- = slight disadvantage
0 = neutral ? = information not available Rx = treatment	

	Standard Option #1	Standard Option #2	Investig. Option #1	Investig. Option #2	No Rx
Remission rate (cancer undetectable after Rx)					- - - -
Duration of remission					- - - -
Response rate (cancer improved after Rx)					- - - -
Cure rate					- - - -
Short-term risks of Rx (infection, heart disease, bleeding, death, etc.)					
Long-term risks of Rx (second cancers, heart disease, osteoporosis, etc.)					
Limits other Rx options (other options too risky or less effective after Rx)					
Length of Rx course					
Effect of Rx on work/home					
Your costs (medications, travel, child care, etc.)					

Don't worry about getting the ratings exact. As you fill in all the boxes, you can adjust the entries you filled in earlier. When done, you'll see a lot of pluses and minuses, and possibly some question marks in the grid. Use the pattern of pluses and minuses to help you rank your treatment options from best to worst. Ideally, after you've filled in the grid, your best treatment choice will be obvious to you. At the very least, Harpham's Decision Tool will help you know what to ask about each of your treatment options, understand your options more clearly, and narrow down your choices to the best two or three.

How do I find out the ratings for each type of treatment?

You assign ratings from ++++ (big advantage) to ---- (big disadvantage) based on accurate information from reliable sources such as your oncologists, the medical literature, and reputable cancer organizations. For purposes of this decision-making tool, ratings must not be based on anecdotal stories, your intuition, or your sense of hopefulness about each treatment. Harpham's Decision Tool is only as useful as the accuracy of the information you use to assign the ratings. Be sure to review your filled-in grid with your physicians.

Can I make changes to Harpham's Decision Tool?

Absolutely! This tool is a model, and the categories and ratings are just suggestions. You may use it exactly as pictured or modify it to suit your personal situation, values, and risk-taking preferences. You may want to put the exact name of the treatments in the top line. Or, when filling in the grid, you may prefer to call them "Option A," "Option B," and so on. You may want to add additional categories such as "Close to Home" or "Preserves Fertility" if being treated near your hometown or maximizing your chance of having your own children in the future is a high priority for you.

Why do some spaces have question marks in them?

When newer treatments and investigational treatments are options for you, some information may not yet be available. For example, new treatments don't have information on cure rates or long-term risks until enough time has transpired since these treatments first came into clinical use. Harpham's Decision Tool will help take these limitations into account as you figure out the best treatment based on the most accurate and up-to-date information available to you today.

How can I make such an important decision based on incomplete information?

One of the hardest things about making a treatment decision is that you have the disease now, and some information about your treatment choices may not be available for years. The best you can do is the best you can do. Don't despair. Doing your best *will* help you. When you methodically and thoughtfully choose a course of treatment, you have reason for real hope.

Why aren't alternative therapies for curing cancer included in Harpham's Decision Tool?

No alternative therapy has been proven effective against cancer. All conventional cancer therapies and all therapies administered in phase-III clinical trials have been proven effective against cancer. If you want to stack the odds in your favor, you'll consider only treatments that have been proven effective.

Why aren't temporary side effects of cancer treatment included in the grid?

It is assumed that you are willing to deal with temporary treatment-related side effects and discomforts that are not health- or life-threatening. Your physicians and nurses can tell you which side effects are common with each type of cancer treatment.

If I know I want to treat my cancer, why should I include a "No Rx" (no treatment) column?

In the process of making a wise treatment decision, you must think about all the risks and uncertainties associated with each option. You may feel frightened or discouraged by the idea of taking on risks and problems that you'd rather avoid. The "no treatment" column serves as a reference to help you keep a healthy perspective. In choosing a course of treatment, you are trading the risks and problems of untreated cancer (note all the minuses in the first four categories of the "no treatment" column) for the risks and problems of treatment.

When treatment is recommended, the overall risks of your untreated cancer are greater than the risks of your proposed treatment.

What if I want to avoid getting toxic treatment and wait for newer, less toxic treatments to become available?

It's understandable if you don't want to expose your body to toxic treatment, especially since you can't go back and unexpose yourself. You may want to delay toxic treatments in the hope that new treatments may become available that are equally effective but less toxic. The problem is this: If you delay effective treatment in the hope of avoiding the associated toxicity, you may die of your cancer while waiting for new treatments to become available.

What if I get flustered or upset when I think about choosing treatment?

Seek out the advice of people who can help you gain the confidence needed to weigh your options and make a decision:

- Your primary-care physician
- A social worker, preferably one trained in oncology social work
- A member of the clergy, particularly someone trained in oncology chaplaincy

What should I do with Harpham's Decision Tool once I've made my final treatment decision?

Put it away and forget about it! It's time to shift gears. Harpham's Decision Tool helps you stack the odds in your favor. Once you've done that, it's time to focus your energies on helping your treatments work. Nourish hope that you will have a good outcome from your treatment.

Why don't I feel 100 percent sure about my final decision regarding treatment?

You may feel unsure about your treatment choice despite having given it your best effort. One reason may be the sense of urgency in making your decision. Even if you had a few weeks to decide without jeopardizing your health, you may feel a sense of time pressure forcing you to make a decision before you feel ready.

Chances are that even with all the time in the world, you would feel a lingering sense of uncertainty. Your qualms may reflect the fact that you must base one of the most important decisions of your life on statistics and uncertainties. No amount of research or bargaining gives you a guarantee that you'll do well and land on the good side of the statistics for your disease and treatment. You can't know for sure that you have made the "right" decision until many years from now. Nor does treatment come with a warranty that any damage can be fixed if you suffer some complication. Unlike a broken car, which you can fix again and again, or trade in if a repair doesn't work, you cannot always fix the damage to your body, and you can never trade in your body for a new one. Few other decisions you make have these kinds of stakes.

You may become unsettled by stories of people with the same type of cancer receiving different treatment. It doesn't make sense to compare yourself with other people unless you know all the details about their situation. Even then, too many unmeasurable factors affect your course, making you different from everyone else.

Last, the treatment you choose may involve physical discomforts, time off from work or school, significant inconveniences, financial strain, and emotional stress. It is hard to choose something that involves physical and emotional distress, especially if you feel fine right now or if there hasn't been time for the reality of your illness to sink in.

Take comfort in the knowledge that you and your physicians are making the wisest decision you can at this time. Once the final decision has been made and you have started treatment, do not look back. Devote your energy toward your treatment.

SUPPORTIVE THERAPIES

What are supportive therapies?

Supportive therapies are conventional treatments that are not directed against cancer cells but are used to help make the cancer treatments safer and more effective, or they help you feel well and regain your health. In this book, the term "supportive therapies" refers to *doctor-prescribed treatments* such as blood products and **growth factors**, nutritional support, oxygen, antibiotics, pain management, antinausea (**antiemetic**) medications, psychological counseling, and rehabilitation. Supportive therapies help prevent, minimize, or treat conditions such as **anemia**, bleeding, infection, heart failure, nausea and vomiting, anxiety, depression, itching, **lymphedema** (swelling of a limb), or breathing difficulties. In helping prevent and treat these side effects and complications, they often help you feel better. "Supplemental therapies," those therapies that can be pursued without a doctor's prescription, are discussed on page 80.

What are growth factors?

Growth factors stimulate normal blood cells to grow, and they may be helpful when blood counts (white blood cells, red blood cells, or **platelets**) are low because of cancer and/or treatments. Low blood counts don't always need to be treated. Before the advent of genetically engineered growth factors, anemia (low red-blood-cell counts) and low platelet counts were treated with blood transfusions when necessary.

What are colony-stimulating factors?

Granulocyte **colony-stimulating factors** (G-CSF) and granulocyte macrophage colony-stimulating factors (GM-CSF) stimulate the bone marrow to make more white blood cells. Given as injections, these growth factors have been shown to be safe and effective tools for shortening the time to recovery of white-blood-cell counts lowered by cancer treatment. Studies are under way to determine in which medical situations the benefits outweigh the risks and expense. Some of these studies are looking at quality-of-life issues such as the ability to work or care for one's family, as well as cost-effectivene factors such as decreased hospitalizations for fever or **sepsis** (blood infection).

What is erythropoietin (EPO)?

Erythropoietin may be helpful in certain cases of anemia by stimulating red-blood-cell production. EPO is expensive, especially when used long-term, but is cost-effective when it offsets frequent blood transfusions and improves quality of life such as by boosting the patient's energy. A longer-lasting form of the drug, darbepoietin, has recently received FDA approval. Not everyone with anemia responds to EPO. Current research is clarifying when it is appropriate to prescribe a course of EPO.

What is thrombopoietin (TPO)?

Thrombopoietin stimulates the production of platelets, the blood cells that play a vital role in clotting. Certain types of cancer and treatment can cause low platelet counts, which puts the patient at risk of bleeding. The development of a safe and effective preparation of thrombopoietin has lagged behind that for colony-stimulating factors and erythropoietin.

What are dendritic cells?

Dendritic cells are also called the most powerful "antigen-presenting cells" (APC). They are immune cells that stimulate other cells in your immune system to recognize and kill cancer cells. Dendritic cells are receiving much attention in research circles not only in terms of understanding how cancer cells outsmart the body's defense systems but also in developing more effective cancer therapies such as vaccines.

What are cytoprotective agents?

Cytoprotective or chemoprotective agents are given to protect normal cells from the damaging effects of cancer therapies. Only a few such agents are currently available.

- Amifostine (Ethyol) helps protect the kidneys from cisplatin-based therapies in patients with head and neck cancer. It may decrease the cumulative nerve and blood toxicity, too.
- Dexrazoxane (Zinecard) helps decrease the incidence and severity of heart damage from doxorubicin (Adriamycin) when given under certain circumstances.
- Leukovorin is used to rescue cells from high doses of methotrexate.
- Mesna is used to help protect the bladder from high doses of cyclophosphamide (Cytoxan) or isophosphamide (Ifosfamide).

What is nutritional support?

Nutritional support is treatment aimed at preventing or reversing malnutrition. Most evidence suggests that being well nourished confers an advantage in fighting disease and tolerating anticancer treatments. A growing trend is under way to prevent malnutrition in patients at risk due to their disease and/or treatments, and to treat those who have evidence of malnutrition. If you can't get adequate nutrients from your diet because of your medical condition, nutritional support may be prescribed. When your digestive tract is working, drinking high-calorie liquid supplements is the preferred approach because of the ease, low risk (when prescribed by professionals), cost-effectiveness, and beneficial effects on the gut (the intestines). Sometimes your digestive system doesn't work and your body is unable to absorb nutrients from any food put in your mouth or directly into your stomach. In this case, total parenteral nutrition (TPN) may be given intravenously, usually through a catheter that empties into a large vein near your heart (see catheters, page 94).

How do I know if I need nutritional support?

Malnutrition is a condition that is determined through a variety of measurements such as skin thickness and blood protein levels. Many cancer patients who are malnourished do not look thin. A physical examination, blood tests, and urine tests can help determine whether you are losing muscle mass or have developed vitamin deficiencies. It is better to treat malnutrition early, before it causes medical problems. No matter what your nutritional status, eating a nutrient-rich diet will help you get and feel better.

What is rehabilitation?

Rehabilitation is therapy aimed at preventing or reversing impairments and disabilities due to your cancer or its treatment. Many therapies that have been successful in improving the condition of people who have suffered a stroke or trauma can help people with similar medical problems due to cancer. For example, if nerve injury or loss of muscle impairs movement of your arm or leg, rehabilitation may help you regain use of your limb. Rehabilitation may be an important element of your pain-management program, too. Interventions include therapeutic exercises, gait training, orthopedic appliances such as leg braces, **prostheses** (artificial body parts), lymphedema treatments, bowel and bladder retraining, speech and swallowing therapy, and occupational therapies.

How do I know if I need rehabilitation?

With everyone focused on your cancer, the opportunity to improve your situation with appropriate rehabilitation may be neglected. If you can no longer perform your usual activities or your treatment is expected to cause impairment, ask your physician about obtaining a consultation from specialists in rehabilitation. (Pain management, diet, and exercise are discussed more fully in chapter 3. Chapter 5 is devoted to dealing with the emotional issues.)

ALTERNATIVE THERAPIES

What are "alternative therapies for curing cancer"?

Alternative (also called unconventional or unorthodox) **therapies** are treatments that are taken by patients *instead* of conventional medical therapy *to control or cure cancer.* These therapies are practiced outside mainstream medicine.

Alternative therapies are not the same as investigational or experimental, or supplemental or complementary therapies. Alternative therapies may claim to be safer, less toxic, and more effective, but *no alternative therapy has been shown scientifically to cure cancer.* Many have been shown to be ineffective at best and possibly harmful, and are often expensive. The National Center for Complementary and Alternative Medicine classified them into seven categories:

- Diet and nutrition (e.g., macrobiotics, megavitamins)
- Bioelectromagnetics
- Alternative-medicine systems (e.g., Chinese medicine, Ayurvedic medicine, homeopathy)
- Pharmacologic and biological therapies (e.g., Burzynski's anti-neoplastons, shark cartilage)
- Manual healing (e.g., therapeutic touch)
- Herbal medicines
- Mind-body techniques (meditation, relaxation)

What are the downsides of alternative therapies for curing cancer?

By definition, no alternative therapy has been proven to be effective against cancer in people. In contrast, every conventional therapy has been scientifically proven to be effective against cancer in people. In other words, with measurable reliability conventional therapy can cure some cancers and prolong life with others.

Alternative therapies can hurt you when they are used instead of conventional therapy because:

- You may miss an opportunity to control or cure your cancer with effective conventional therapy if you spend critical time investigating or taking alternative therapy.
- You can get a false sense of security that you are being treated and followed adequately when in fact you are not.
- You may be taking unnecessary risks associated with the therapy.
- You may spend a lot of money, especially since insurance companies rarely reimburse for alternative therapies (note the long, well-documented history of charlatans taking advantage of patients—a problem that continues today).

If you are taking conventional cancer therapy, the addition of certain unconventional cancer therapies may increase the risks or decrease the effectiveness of your conventional therapies.

What about the stories documenting cures with alternative therapy?

Testimonials abound documenting the effectiveness of alternative therapies for curing cancer. Though exciting and inspiring, they do not constitute scientific evidence. Anecdotes offer no way of proving that the treatment was responsible in any way for the patient's improvement or cure. In many cases, the patient also took conventional therapy. Even if an alternative therapy did help some individual(s), there is no way to know if the same therapy offers *you* any benefit.

It's too easy to get a skewed view. Proponents of alternative therapies often omit mentioning the lack of scientific proof. Publishers of books and magazines know that failure stories don't sell well, so they rarely print stories by or about the many people who took the same alternative treatments without benefit (or who were harmed, or died). Patients who feel they made a mistake by taking alternative therapies may keep their experience a secret out of embarrassment, shame, or desire to put it all behind them.

The National Institutes of Health (NIH) have established the Office of Alternative Medicine to assess scientifically the value of various alternative therapies. Some alternative therapies already have been tested and have proven to be ineffective and/or harmful to patients with cancer. Most alternative therapies have not been subjected to rigorous scientific study. Until these studies are done, it is irresponsible to label or promote an untested alternative therapy as a treatment for curing cancer. Keep in mind that people have been using so-called alternative treatments for thousands of years. Yet, only in the past few decades have large numbers of people with cancer been cured or enjoyed long survival, and this survivorship is due to advances in mainstream science and technology.

What if I feel that alternative therapy is a good cancer treatment?

Many factors make alternative therapies for curing cancer attractive. You may:

- Find the risks and side effects of conventional therapy more frightening than the alternative therapies that are portrayed as pain-free and nontoxic.
- Feel discouraged because your cancer is difficult to cure or treat, and conventional doctors tell you that they can't guarantee success. The doctors involved with alternative therapy may seem to be more optimistic and/or more supportive. They may tell you that they are offering you a cure, which is, of course, what you want to hear.
- Have had unpleasant experiences with conventional medical doctors in the past, which makes it harder for you to communicate with or trust conventional oncologists. Or, you may find the setting of alternative medicine more soothing and personal than the offices and hospitals of conventional medicine.
- Feel pressured by well-intentioned friends and family to look into alternative therapies. You may want to avoid disappointing others or causing social tension.
- Be overwhelmed by your diagnosis and find it hard to know what to believe or do.

One of the most important decisions you will make is what treatments you take to control or cure your cancer. If you proceed with treatment that is ineffective or harmful, you will lose valuable time that could make a major difference for your future.

How can I recognize quackery?

There are warning signs of possible **quackery**. Beware if the company, clinic, or person offering treatment

- claims the treatment is harmless, painless, and nontoxic;
- uses a secret formula that is never revealed and cannot be tested or reproduced by anyone else;
- explains the treatment's action on the basis of unproven theories;
- requires patients to follow special diets or intense nutritional support during and after treatment (in which case the failure

of the treatment can be blamed on the patient's inability to follow the rigorous diet);
- discusses their treatment only in the mass media;
- supports the success of their treatments with testimonials and anecdotes;
- has never done controlled studies to document effectiveness;
- is not staffed by certified cancer specialists;
- does not require a consent form;
- attacks the medical establishment.

Is there any role for alternative therapy in the treatment of cancer?

The National Cancer Institute (NCI) defines alternative therapy as that which is taken *instead of* conventional therapy. If you have any conventional treatment options, these give you a better chance of cure and longer life than any alternative therapy.

You may be interested in using an unconventional cancer treatment *along with* your conventional cancer treatments. The NCI defines these unconventional therapies as *complementary* therapies (see page 80). Obtain objective, scientific information about the risks and benefits to you of combining any unconventional therapy with your conventional cancer treatments. In particular, you need to ensure that the unconventional therapy you are considering will not counteract or interfere with your conventional therapy.

If you have faith in the ability of an unconventional therapy to kill your cancer cells, and if all your doctors feel that it poses no additional risk, you may decide to take this unconventional therapy along with the recommended conventional cancer therapies. This approach allows you to pursue options that you feel are beneficial, and helps you to regain a sense of control, without depriving you of the benefits of conventional medicine.

Make sure you know how the word "alternative" is being used when referring to a specific therapy. Many people use the term "alternative therapy" for *any* treatment that is not practiced in mainstream medicine whether used *instead of* or *with* conventional therapies, and whether used to cure cancer or just to feel better in some way. In this context, nontraditional healing techniques that are used in addition to conventional cancer therapy, especially to relieve side effects or stress, may have a role in your treatment and are discussed more fully in the section on supplementary therapies on page 80.

Discuss your findings with your oncologist before you make your final decision about which cancer treatments to pursue.

What is integrative medicine?

Practitioners who combine conventional cancer therapies with selected unconventional complementary therapies are said to be practicing integrative medicine.

Can I use any unconventional cancer treatments when I'm in a clinical trial?

Probably not. Every patient has to be taking as close to the same treatments as possible in order for reliable conclusions to be derived about the treatments being tested in the study. If you decide to receive investigational cancer therapy in a clinical trial and you want to use an unconventional treatment, too, be sure to ask your doctors if this is okay.

What if my oncologist discourages me from taking unconventional cancer therapies?

It is best if everything you do on your own to try to control your cancer is under the auspices of your oncologist so that your progress can be monitored, problems can be detected and treated, and any benefits of conventional therapy are not offset. If your oncologist adamantly opposes your pursing unconventional therapies along with your conventional medicines, and if you feel that you must do both, it is safest for you to find a reputable oncologist who feels comfortable with your proposed treatments. If you can't, the next best situation is for your oncologist to be aware of what you are doing, even if he or she disagrees with your choice.

You are taking a risk when you don't keep your doctors informed about all the therapies that you are pursuing.

Treatments given to cure or control cancer cells include:

• **Conventional** (mainstream; standard)
Treatment used widely in American cancer centers. *All conventional therapies have been proven to be effective against cancer.* Even when conventional therapy doesn't offer a cure for your type of cancer, it often can delay the progression of your cancer and improve your quality of life by minimizing medical complications such as pain, chemical imbalances, malnutrition, anxiety, and depression.
    Examples: standard doses of chemotherapy, radiation therapy, or biologic therapy.

• **Investigational** (experimental)
Treatments administered in clinical trials. In phase-III trials, the treatment under investigation is known to be effective against cancer; the study is set up to determine how it compares to standard therapy. In phase-I and -II trials, effectiveness is unknown; however, these trials are based on preclinical studies and are done only with patients for whom there is no effective standard therapy available.

• **Alternative** (unconventional; unorthodox)
Treatment that is designed and administered outside mainstream conventional medicine. *No alternative therapy has been proven scientifically to be effective against cancer.* If you want to optimize your chance for recovery, don't use alternative cancer treatments instead of effective standard treatments that should be administered now.
    Examples: laetrile (apricot pit medicine), macrobiotics, homeopathy, Chinese herbal remedies, laying on of hands.

(Note: When an unconventional therapy for curing cancer is used in addition to conventional cancer therapy, it is called "complementary therapy." To complicate matters more, the term "complementary" is often used in reference to both conventional and unconventional supplemental therapies.)

Treatments given to help the body stay as healthy or comfortable as possible (i.e., not intended to kill cancer cells) include:

- **Supportive** (conventional supportive; standard supportive)
  These conventional treatments are used in mainstream medicine to decrease the risks of cancer and conventional cancer treatments.
  Examples: colony-stimulating factors, intravenous nutritional support, oxygen, antibiotics.

- **Conventional supplementary** (standard complementary; adjunctive; supplementary; complementary)
  These treatments are usually available through clinics and hospitals that practice conventional medicine, and are intended to help improve quality of life.
  Examples: psychological or spiritual counseling or support, nutritional counseling, exercise programs, massage, relaxation, visualization.

- **Unconventional supplementary** (alternative supplementary; complementary supplementary; supplementary complementary)
  These treatments are available through clinics and hospitals that practice unconventional medicine.
  Examples: vitamin supplementation, homeopathy, therapeutic touch.

What if I am too embarrassed to tell my doctors that I am thinking about or already using an unconventional therapy?

Many people fear scorn or rejection by their doctors if they choose to follow unconventional cancer treatments such as macrobiotic diets or healing touch. Keeping your doctors informed of everything you are doing to treat your cancer allows them to

- reassure you when these measures are safe;
- give you solid reasons why an unconventional diet or treatment could cause you problems;
- adjust your conventional therapies, as needed.

Oncologists know that many patients look at or use unconventional therapies. Sharing information with your doctors maximizes the safety of the treatments they prescribe. If your oncologists disapprove of your unconventional therapies, they still will be able to take better care of you because they are aware of what you are doing. You may have to seek the care of another oncologist if your current oncologists feel that they cannot take good care of you while you are also taking specific unconventional therapy that they feel is dangerous. A doctor-patient relationship is built on trust. You owe it to yourself and to your doctors to be honest.

How can I tell if a treatment is conventional or alternative, or supplementary or complementary?

The many terms used to describe treatments are confusing, and different people (including experts) use the various terms differently. To make matters worse, there is overlap in some of the definitions. For example, homeopathy is considered alternative if used *instead of* conventional cancer therapies and it is considered complementary if used *with* them. Acupuncture, when used to control nausea or pain, is considered conventional by some physicians and unconventional by others. Be sure that you understand how each term is being used when describing your treatment choices. In particular, *be sure you know whether the treatment is intended to treat your cancer* or to help your body stay as healthy or comfortable as possible while other treatment is aimed at the cancer. Find out what is known about the risks and benefits of each treatment.

It is straightforward whether a particular treatment prescribed to treat cancer cells is conventional or not. You can find out by asking your physicians or calling the Cancer Information Service (1-800-4-CANCER).

SUPPLEMENTAL THERAPIES

What are supplemental therapies?

Supplemental therapies, also called adjunctive therapies or **complementary therapies**, are treatments used in mainstream medicine that are intended to promote your physical and emotional comfort, enhance your response to conventional therapy, and speed your recovery from treatment. Supplemental therapies are used *in addition* to the conventional therapy that is aimed at the cancer cells, and most are available without a prescription. Some proponents believe that they also improve your chances against your cancer. Examples include visual imagery, music therapy, massage therapy, special diets, prayer, humor, biofeedback, meditation, exercise, and relaxation techniques. Supplemental therapy should never be used as your *only* cancer therapy when effective anticancer therapy is available.

(Note that the terms "supplementary" and "complementary" often are used interchangeably when referring to any therapy that is not aimed at the cancer.)

Who prescribes supplemental therapies?

Most supplemental therapies are not prescribed in the usual sense of the word. In fact, your oncologists may never even mention supplemental therapies unless you ask specific questions about them. Counselors in oncology, psychologists and psychiatrists, social workers, and licensed therapists are the professionals in mainstream medicine who most often evaluate patients and recommend supplemental therapies. You should discuss any proposed therapies with your oncologists before you begin, especially if you are going to put anything into your body such as special foods or pills.

What are the disadvantages of supplemental therapy?

Each supplemental therapy has advantages and disadvantages. On the one hand, when you believe in the potential benefit of a particular supplemental therapy, you nourish hope and regain a sense of control. On the other hand, if you feel pressured to pursue supplemental therapies, or if you want to believe but actually are skeptical of the benefits, the pursuit may be counterproductive. Under these and other circumstances, various supplemental therapies heighten rather than lessen anxiety, drain rather than bolster energy, and cause rather than relieve symptoms.

The use of supplemental therapy requires an investment of your time, energy, and, often, money. Even though most are nonprescription, some may involve a real risk of significant physical or emotional harm, especially since your body is dealing with the stress of cancer. Find out from knowledgeable people (doctors, nurses, social workers, and counselors) what your options are. Discuss the potential benefits and risks to you as indicated by reliable data. Information about supplemental therapy will allow you to maximize the use of the various worthy resources that can assist your personal healing.

How quickly do I need to make a decision about the use of any supplemental therapies?

Decisions about supplemental therapies do not carry the same urgency or weight as those about your anticancer treatments. If you feel overwhelmed by information and decision making right now, think about supplemental therapies later. If you are taking a supplemental therapy and change your mind about its value to you, usually you can stop it. If you decide you'd like to start one that your doctors agree is safe, usually you can begin at any time.

What about complementary therapies?

Unconventional therapies that are given to reduce stress or side effects of cancer treatment or to enhance the body's ability to fight cancer are called complementary therapies. Although often presented in scientific-sounding language, only a small proportion of these therapies have been subjected to scientific evaluation.

Some unconventional complementary therapies are safe; others are dangerous. Some unconventional complementary therapies are used by conventional practitioners in an integrative approach to treating cancer. Other complementary therapies are rarely, if ever, used in integrative medicine because they are considered unsafe and/or ineffective.

As with any other medical procedure or treatment, before you agree to use a specific complementary treatment, you need to find out

• if it might diminish the safety or effectiveness of your cancer therapies;

- the risks and benefits to someone with your type of cancer in your situation;
- the credentials and experience of the prescribing practitioner;
- the costs.

(As mentioned earlier, some people also refer to conventional therapies used to reduce stress or side effects of cancer treatment or to enhance the body's ability to fight cancer as "complementary.")

Cancer and its treatment are risky and difficult enough. Be sure to avoid any complementary therapies that might make your conventional cancer therapy less effective or cause additional problems.

What are antioxidants?

When cells are damaged, so-called reactive oxygen species (ROS), or free radicals, are released. These ROS can damage normal cells and are believed to play a role in the development of cancer in healthy people. ROS also are involved in the development of certain side effects and late effects of cancer therapies, such as neuropathy and scarring. **Antioxidants** are substances that mop up these free radicals and thus protect healthy cells from their damaging effects. Examples of antioxidants include beta-carotene, selenium, shark cartilage, viamin C, vitamin E, and carotenoids.

How will my taking supplemental antioxidants affect my cancer therapy?

It depends! One theory suggests that antioxidants increase the ability of conventional therapies to destroy cancer cells. An opposing theory suggests that supplemental antioxidants make conventional cancer therapy less effective. Most research that has been done on animals and in people suggest that antioxidant supplements can be *helpful* or *harmful*.

Whether supplemental antioxidants will help or harm *you* will depend on

- the specific type and stage of your cancer;
- specifics regarding your metabolism;
- the presence or absence of other conditions, your use of other medications;
- the exact type of conventional cancer treatment you are receiving;
- the exact type and amount of antioxidant supplement being considered;
- factors that are still unclear.

Recent studies are giving very mixed results. In some cases, the use of specific supplements by patients with specific types of cancer has been associated with worse outcomes, presumably because the supplemental antioxidants protected the cancer cells from the damaging effects of conventional cancer therapy. In other cases, when patients had different cancer situations and/or used different supplements, outcomes appear better.

Unless reputable oncologists have shown that a particular supplemental antioxidant is safe and effective for someone like you, you risk worsening your outcome by taking supplements.

What about the use of supplemental antioxidants in the prevention of side effects or late effects of conventional cancer treatments?

Studies are under way to see if supplemental antioxidants can prevent side effects or late effects of radiation or chemotherapy. Hopefully, answers will be forthcoming about which antioxidants are safe and effective for treating which patients. Until research is done regarding a particular supplement, in a specific dose, given to patients just like you, any potential role of supplemental antioxidants in your care remains unclear.

What if I want to take supplemental antioxidants?

Before you take any supplements, talk with your doctors. Find out if they might decrease the effectiveness of your therapy or increase your chance of complications. If you want the health benefits of antioxidants, instead of using supplements that have not been proven safe and effective, include antioxidant-rich fruits and vegetables in your daily diet (after getting your physicians' approval).

First do no harm! Use supplements only if you and your oncologist have discussed and determined them to be safe for you.

What is visualization?

Visualization is the process of imagining a desired effect or outcome in your mind. Athletes, actors, and other performers use this technique successfully to enhance their performances. Many patients learn how to visualize their body healing. You can use graphic realistic mental images of white cells killing cancer cells. You might prefer using symbols such as white dots gobbling up blue dots to represent your white cells destroying your cancer cells. Visualization can be very abstract, too. For example, the image of an ocean wave washing over a beach and then retreating to the ocean carrying away debris might help you imagine your cancer treatment and immune system getting rid of your cancer cells.

What is the role of visualization in healing and in fighting cancer?

Visualization does help some people with problems such as pain, migraine headaches, insomnia, and muscle spasm. No study to date on people with cancer has shown any significant effect on response or cure rates, or rates of cancer recurrence. However, it helps some patients gain confidence or relax. It is a safe and relatively inexpensive tool (although audiotapes for assisting in visualization aren't always cheap) for people in whom it helps alleviate physical and emotional symptoms. As for your cancer, visualization can't make it worse, and it can help decrease negative stress by giving you some sense of control.

Visualization is counterproductive if you feel guilty when you don't do it or feel responsible if you have medical problems despite genuine efforts to visualize. There is no one right way to visualize, and visualization is not for everyone.

What about hypnosis?

Hypnosis can be a safe and effective way to help control pain, nausea, anxiety, or other unpleasant side effects of cancer and cancer therapy. Professionals trained in hypnosis can teach you to achieve a state of relaxed consciousness so that your subconscious is more susceptible to helpful suggestion (e.g., "I will be hungry for lunch after I finish today's chemotherapy"; "I will be calm when I go for my CT scan"). With time, patients learn to achieve this state on their own through self-hypnosis. Hypnosis can be thought of as an extension of self-relaxation, biofeedback, visual imagery, or meditation.

People may be reluctant to consider hypnosis because of their notion of a magician using hypnosis to levitate a subject, or a psychiatrist using it to release a patient's painful repressed memories. In modern, practical terms, hypnosis is a simple technique that enables you to have more control over your body's functions. Make sure that the hypnotist, oftentimes a psychiatrist, is well trained in this skill.

What about the role of humor?

Cancer is serious business, but you don't have to be sad or serious *all the time*. Genuine laughter offers physical and psychological benefits in a pleasurable way. Comedy can give you a break from problems, relieve tension between you and others, lighten oppressive circumstances, and help you regain a sense of control.

Try putting humor into your daily routine. Look for or create situations or images that tickle your funny bone: Watch *Blooper* videos, read comics or funny books, share jokes or puns. Try keeping a humor diary in which you record situations, cartoons, jokes, anecdotes, or things you see or hear that strike you as funny. Then pull out your diary on days when you need a lift.

Let your friends and family know that it is okay for them to be happy when they can, even if you're having a hard day. Humor can be a powerful ally as long as you (and your family and friends) use it in ways that are comfortable for you, and as long as joking around doesn't keep you from getting good medical care.

Where can I find out more about humor and healing?

You can call or write for the quarterly newsletter of the Association for Applied and Therapeutic Humor: 1951 W. Camelback Rd. Ste. 445, Phoenix AZ 85015; telephone 602-995-1454, FAX 602-995-1449, office@aath.org. Another starting point can be The HUMOR Project, Inc., 110 Spring St., Saratoga Springs, NY 12866; 518-587-8770.

How quickly does my treatment need to be started?

If you are having symptoms from your cancer or you have a very fast-growing cancer, then you will probably need to get started on treatment quickly. If you were diagnosed by a biopsy of a painless lump, you probably have some time to make your decision. Your doctors will be able to advise you about how much time you have to decide on therapy.

Cancer therapy is a big commitment in terms of time, energy, emotions, and money. Once you get started, you can never turn back the clock, erase the effects of whatever treatment you've already received, and try again as if you're starting over. Your body may be different after treatments, whether the treatments worked or not. Your cancer may be different, too, after having been exposed to treatments. It is wise to invest the time and energy into researching with your doctor what is the best treatment plan *for you*, a conclusion that usually depends on the results of adequate staging. Keep in mind that your cancer will continue to grow until treatment is started. If you spend too much time delaying or researching, you may be losing valuable and irretrievable treatment time.

Cancer treatment is your way to improved health and well-being.

Once you've decided on a course of treatment, the next chapter will help you learn how to manage the medical problems so that you can get through your treatments as safely and comfortably as possible.

3

Managing the Practical Problems

It's one thing to make wise treatment choices; it's quite another to live with them and to support them with proper action. This chapter will teach you how to be an effective cancer patient—knowing when to call the doctor, what to do about your diet or exercise program, how to cope with pain and fatigue, and where to go for help.

GENERAL MEDICAL CONCERNS

How do I know when to call the doctor with a question or problem and when to wait until my scheduled visit?

In general, if you feel that a symptom or change in your condition *might* be important, call your doctors' office or answering service. If you are spending time and energy trying to decide whether or not to call, or you find yourself trying not to worry about something you've noticed, pick up the phone and make the call. Your oncologists do not expect you to know exactly what can wait and what needs immediate attention.

It's better to sound a false alarm than to have a treatable problem go unattended. Many medical problems are easier to fix when they are small or at an early stage. An infection or chemical imbalance may be easy to treat if addressed at the inconvenient hour of 2 A.M. If left untreated until the more respectable hour of 8 A.M., these complications may end up requiring in-hospital care and could threaten your life.

For what specific problems should I call my doctor?

Call your doctor for:

- Fever. Ask your doctor or nurse which temperature guidelines to use. When blood counts are down, even low-grade fevers become important. Certain cancers, however, cause fevers that do not need to be reported every time they occur.
- Shaking chills
- New signs or symptoms (*new* rash, pain, severe headache, swelling, shortness of breath, numbness or weakness of any part of the body)
- A worsening of an old sign or symptom
- Inability to keep down fluids or medicines
- Bleeding or unusual bruising
- Increasing or uncontrolled pain

Even when you have been forewarned to expect a problem, notify your doctor's office if

- the problem seems worse than you expected;
- the problem is lasting longer than you expected;
- medicines given to treat the problem aren't working well; or
- you are quite uncomfortable.

If I do not have many side effects, is my therapy still working?

Yes. Many people have few or no significant side effects from their therapy, and their cancer melts away.

Do people ever stop their treatment before it is completed?

Yes. If problems come up during your therapy (such as intolerable side effects, medical complications, or a poor response of your cancer), your physician will reassess your situation and consider switching you to a different therapy. If a newer treatment with clear advantages should become available during your therapy, this can be considered for you, too.

How should I proceed if I am due for a routine test having nothing to do with my cancer?

Contact your regular doctors to be sure they are aware of your cancer diagnosis, evaluation, and treatment plans. Discuss with your regular doctors *and* your oncologist whether you should proceed with a routine test or procedure, such as a mammogram, stress test, colon exam, skin exam, gynecology exam, routine complete physical, and so on (dental examinations are discussed on page 100). Some screening tests are part of your cancer workup and need to be done now anyway. If your doctors advise that you proceed with a test, discuss who should order the test (namely, your regular doctors or your oncologist).

Some tests can be safely postponed, and delaying them allows you to devote your energy and attention to taking care of your cancer. Some tests should not be done now, either because they will not give reliable results or because they are not as safe given your current condition or treatment. Occasionally a routine screening test becomes urgent in light of your cancer diagnosis. Any time a doctor advises a test or procedure, be sure to discuss your cancer before anything is done.

How should I proceed if I was due for a routine visit with another doctor for follow-up of a chronic medical condition?

Notify your oncologist when you are due for a medical or dental follow-up of conditions unrelated to your cancer, such as high blood pressure, diabetes, and heart and kidney disease. Your cancer and cancer therapy may affect your other medical conditions. In addition, staying on top of these conditions may help minimize medical problems that can affect your cancer treatments. Sometimes your checkup with your oncologist can replace your checkup with your regular doctor. Usually you will need to continue your routine visits with your regular doctor *in addition* to your visits to your oncologist for your cancer.

Be your own best advocate. Keep up with all your checkups, cancer related *and* non–cancer related. Make sure that each doctor who treats you is aware of what the other doctors are doing. Do not hesitate to ask the doctors to communicate with one another if there are any questions or concerns.

What can I expect at my checkups?

Checkups allow your oncologist to

- determine if your treatments are working;
- determine if your treatments are causing any medical problems;
- determine if your next treatment needs to be adjusted in any way (for example, timing or dosage);
- see how you are adjusting to each phase of your illness;
- address your questions and concerns.

Do I have to prepare for my checkups?

In most cases, yes. Working together, you and your doctors can arrive at a plan of action by the end of your visit. Your doctor's job is to evaluate your condition, understand your concerns, and provide information and recommendations. Your job is to describe your problems and concerns as clearly as possible. Most patients do this well with some advance preparation.

You are not expected to be an expert at describing your symptoms and problems, but your checkups will be less stressful if you are prepared. You will be better served, too, because the information you provide will be more accurate and more complete. How many times have you left the doctor's office and realized that you forgot to mention something important?

You may recoil at the idea of preparing a list of questions and problems, feeling that you should not be treated like a car being brought to the shop. Or you may worry that a list would make you look like a hypochondriac. Understandably, you want to feel that you are being treated like a whole person. It's hard when your doctors focus right away on the physical problems, ask countless questions, and never seem to have enough time for explanations or a normal conversation.

Like everyone else, doctors face time constraints. What you may interpret as abruptness may be your doctor's attempt to be organized so that information given is complete and accurate, and so that your most serious problems are addressed. A vague, unstructured discussion or a discussion that focuses on one issue may make you feel better emotionally but divert your doctor from some important considerations. Ironically, the more direct the exchange of information at the beginning of your visit, the more time is left to discuss your emotional and social concerns, to relate socially as two people, and for your doctor to offer comfort and support.

Some doctors appreciate your coming prepared with a list; others may be put off. Just remember (and mention to your doctor, if necessary) that the list is *for you* so that you can keep your thoughts organized.

Your doctors can best care for you through a team effort at understanding and solving your problems.

How can I prepare for my checkups?

Before each visit, make a written list of your concerns and questions in order of their importance to you. Don't leave anything out because what you consider to be minor or insignificant may turn out to be a critical piece of information to your doctor. Think about how to present your information in a concise yet complete way. If there is not enough time to cover everything with your doctor, he or she can glance through your list and spot any potentially serious problems that need to be addressed. Before your visit:

- Make a list of any physical, emotional, or practical problems that you have been experiencing.
- Make a list of your questions about your condition, problems, evaluation, and treatments.
- Know what time you need to arrive at the office.
- Know whether you need to be fasting.

You may find it helpful to bring a friend or family member to your visits. Even at routine checkups when everything is going smoothly, you may not remember everything your doctor says. Bring someone to be a second listener. This will take some of the pressure off you. Also, you may appreciate having a companion to talk to immediately afterward, especially if a change in plans is discussed at the visit.

Why do I have to put on a gown at so many visits?

Hospital gowns enable your doctors and nurses to see, hear, feel, and thus learn more about your body. The more they know about you, the better. Some of your visits will have a physical exam as part of the planned agenda. Other visits will add an examination only after you mention a symptom or concern, or if something unexpected shows up on your test results. It is convenient for you, the staff, and the doctor if you are already in a gown. Being prepared in a gown also maximizes the time that is being devoted to evaluating your condition. Patient gowns are not glamorous or insulated. If you are cold or uncomfortable, ask for a blanket or sweater.

Why do they draw blood at so many visits?

Blood tests are a relatively easy way of getting important information about your cancer and your body's response to treatment. Some cancers, such as leukemia, need close watching to be sure the cancer is not putting you in any new danger. Some treatments, such as chemotherapy, cause changes in your blood that need close monitoring. Shifts in your blood chemistry or blood cells can occur over hours to days, so it is common for people to need blood work regularly during therapy. Some changes are predictable; others are not. Keeping a close eye on you helps your doctors find problems early, when they are easier to treat.

Why do I have to take medicines in my vein (intravenously)?

Medicines taken by mouth, so-called oral therapy (pills and liquids), are an easy and safe way to be treated. However, your doctors may prescribe intravenous therapy because of one or more of the following important advantages over oral therapy:

• Some medications *only* work when given in a vein (for example, when stomach juices inactivate the drug).

- I.V. medications and fluids can be given when you can't eat or when your digestion isn't working normally.
- Some medications are safer or more effective when *exact* levels of the medicine are maintained in your blood—a goal that is better achieved or only possible using the intravenous method.

What is access?

Access refers to a connection between the outside of your body and your bloodstream. Access is needed to:

- Obtain blood samples
- Give medicines such as chemotherapy, pain medicines, antibiotics, antinausea medications, and drugs for your heart or lungs
- Give fluids
- Give blood products
- Give nutrition

Types of access incude:

- Peripheral access: access in a body part far from your heart, most often an I.V.—intravenous line—in your arm
- Central access: access to the big vessels near your heart with a central line **catheter** or port

What is an I.V.?

I.V. stands for intravenous, or "in the vein." "Peripheral access" is a fancy term for the usual I.V. tube, or plastic catheter, which is inserted into your hand or arm. This allows fluids or medications to be given directly into your bloodstream. The big disadvantage is that an I.V. in your arm should be changed every three days or so. Notify your doctor's office if you develop redness, swelling, drainage, or pain around the site where the I.V. is inserted.

What is a PICC line (peripherally inserted central catheter)?

A PICC is a long, soft, hollow tube that is inserted into a vein in the elbow crease and threaded up that vein into a large vein near the heart. It has many of the advantages of a **venous access**

device (see next question). Since it is inserted similarly to an I.V., it has the advantage of avoiding the risks and expense of minor surgery. The main disadvantage is that, like peripheral I.V.'s, it can be used for only a few days.

What is a venous access device (VAD)?

A VAD is an IV that goes into your central circulation near your heart, and can stay in for weeks or months at a time. When you will be needing lengthy treatment, or if your veins are small and hard to use, your doctors may recommmend that you have one of the following types of VAD implanted:

- a central venous access catheter (nontunneled or tunneled)
- a port (a device that is entirely under the skin, see page 97)

What are the advantages of having a venous access device (VAD)?

The advantages are:

- You can give blood samples and receive medicines, fluids, and blood repeatedly without the pain or worry of having to stick a new vein each time.
- Access difficulties are avoided when interruption of therapy is unacceptable, such as when you need intravenous pain management or blood-thinning medicines.
- Some medicines are safer when delivered through a large central vein compared to through a small vein in your arm.
- Your arms and hands are free during therapy
- Ports and some catheters can be left in place for weeks to months.
- The catheter is easy to use and easy to remove.

What is a nontunneled catheter (also called a subclavian catheter, central venous catheter [CVC], or central line)?

This is a soft, hollow plastic tube (catheter) with one tip sitting in a large vein near the heart and the other end resting outside your body with a cap on the end. Since these catheters are not tunneled but are inserted directly into one of the large veins near the

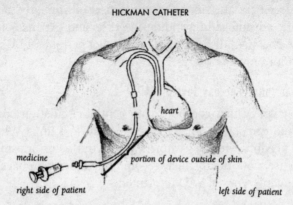

Schematic diagram of a Hickman catheter. Medicine, blood, or fluids can
be injected into the end of the tube that lies outside of the skin. The rest
of the device is under the skin. The catheter ends in or above the right
side of the heart.

heart, they are easier to put in but have a higher risk of infection
and are usable for only a few days. The disadvantages are:

- Slight risk of bleeding or temporary lung collapse
- Inconvenience of caring for the catheter
- Expense of supplies needed to care for the catheter
- Risks of infection or malfunction in the catheter that may
  require catheter removal
- Cosmetic effect of an external catheter

Many times, even when a problem arises with a central venous
catheter, there are ways of solving the problem without removing it.

What is a tunneled catheter?

Broviac or Hickman central venous catheters are "tunneled"
under the skin of the chest wall after the tip has been placed
within a large vein near the heart. Tunneled catheters come in
a wider variety, some having two or three separate channels
(double or triple "lumen"), which allow more than one medication or fluid to be given simultaneously. The main advantage over nontunneled catheters is the decreased risk of

infection that allows the catheter to be used for a long time (weeks or months). The main disadvantage is the minor surgery needed for insertion.

What is involved in caring for a central venous access device?

Central venous catheters must be cared for properly to help prevent infection or blockage due to clotting. You will be taught how to remove old dressings, clean the area where the catheter exits your body, and place a new dressing. After a little bit of practice, most people become adept at caring for their catheters. If you don't feel well enough to handle the care of your **central line**, or you're too squeamish, you can have someone else (such as a close relative or friend) care for it for you until you feel up to it.

What problems can occur with a central venous catheter?

Problems that can occur which require *immediate* attention include:

- Infection signaled by fever and/or chills, or redness, tenderness, pain, drainage, or swelling at the insertion site
- Blood clot formation in the vein signaled by swelling of the face, neck, chest, or arm on the side of the catheter
- Loosening or loss of the cap
- Shortening or lengthening of the catheter
- Leaking catheter

Problems that don't require immediate attention include:

- Itching or skin irritation under the dressing
- Redness around sutures or the insertion site without pain, swelling, or drainage
- Loose or missing sutures

When in doubt regarding your catheter, call your doctor's office.

What is a port?

A venous access **port**, also called an "**implanted port**," is similar to the other central catheters except that the entire device is

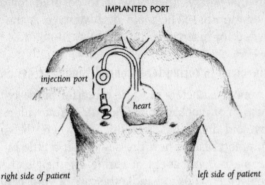

IMPLANTED PORT

injection port

heart

right side of patient

left side of patient

Schematic diagram of an implanted port. The *entire* device is under the
skin. Medicine, blood, or fluids can be injected into the injection port.
Even though the needle goes through the skin into the port, it is a
relatively painless procedure to use this device. There are many
advantages to a totally implantable device.

under the skin. It is inserted while the patient is under general
anesthesia. To get blood, or give blood, fluids, or medicines, a
special needle is inserted through the skin into the implanted
chamber (also called a "reservoir"). Ports

- are easier to use and maintain than external catheters;
- have a lower risk of infection or blockage (clotting);
- are cosmetically preferable (entire device is under the skin).

What is an infusion pump?

Small infusion devices deliver a continuous flow ("infusion") of
medicine into a vein or artery through your intravenous line (I.V.),
central venous catheter (CVC), or implanted port. Pumps allow
patients to be treated as outpatients when they require therapy
that is safer or more effective when given by continuous infusion.
Some pumps are worn like a beeper; others are implanted under
the skin.

How do I know what kind of access device I should have?

There are advantages and disadvantages to each of the many
access devices available. Your doctors can review the best options

for you and advise you which would be the best choice based on your individual circumstances. You may feel a bit overwhelmed at first and want to avoid dealing with anything new. Many people have experienced intravenous treatments both with and without a central line. Most are grateful for the benefits of the catheter and say, "I wish I had done this earlier."

Do I need any vaccinations against infections?

People are more susceptible to infections when they:

- Have certain cancers
- Are receiving some cancer therapies
- Have had their spleen removed

Most vaccinations are given in hopes of building up immunity to specific infectious agents *before* a person is exposed to the illness. After a person's immunity has been boosted by the vaccination, exposure to the infection usually will result in milder illness or no illness at all. Vaccines protect you from only the specific infection covered in the vaccine. There are some risks involved with vaccinations. Discuss with your doctor whether you are a candidate for any vaccinations.

Do I need a pneumonia shot?

The pneumonia shot helps prevent the most common type of pneumonia, pneumococcal pneumonia. You are at increased risk of getting or having complications of pneumococcal infection if:

- Your spleen has been removed.
- Your immune system is weakened by cancer or treatment.

Discuss with your doctor the optimum timing of your vaccination because it takes a few weeks to build up immunity from the vaccination, and the vaccination may not work if given when your immune system is weak. The Centers for Disease Control and Prevention recommends that close contacts (housemates, children, other close associates) of people who need the pneumonia shot also receive the vaccine. This will minimize the chance of a contact bringing the infection to the patient.

Do I need a flu shot?

The flu shot is given every fall (around October) to people at increased risk of influenza. If you have a serious cancer or will be undergoing therapy that will weaken your immune system, ask your doctors about receiving a flu vaccine. Because it takes a few weeks to build up immunity from the vaccination, and it may not work as well if given when your immune system is weak, timing is important. The Centers for Disease Control and Prevention recommends that close contacts (housemates, children, other close associates) of people at increased risk for influenza also receive the vaccine.

Can my children proceed with their routine vaccinations?

Live vaccines are composed of living viruses that have been treated in such a way that they are unable or unlikely to cause serious illness *in healthy people*. If your immune system is weakened by your cancer or cancer treatments, exposure to someone who has recently received a live vaccine may pose a risk to you.

In most cases, the vaccine of concern is the live oral polio vaccine. Discuss your cancer diagnosis and treatments with your children's pediatrician. The pediatrician can tell you if the children's live polio vaccine can be safely delayed until your treatment is complete. Many times, the children will receive the inactivated polio shot which poses no risk to you. Later, they can be given the live vaccine. Their pediatrician and your oncologist can help you balance your children's medical needs against yours.

Do I need a dental exam?

A dental exam, teeth cleaning, and needed periodontal work may be recommended prior to chemotherapy or starting radiation to the head and neck areas. These cancer treatments can increase the chance of dental problems and/or increase the risk associated with treating any problems that arise during the course of therapy for your cancer. Make sure that your dentist knows how you are being treated for your cancer. If any additional dental work is required during the course of your cancer treatment, discuss it with your oncologist before proceeding.

What if my physician tells me to quit smoking or to quit chewing tobacco now? Isn't it too late for that to help?

Quitting cigarettes and smokeless tobacco (chewing tobacco) is one of the most powerful of the many measures you can take to help your body get well again and stay well. Avoiding all tobacco products is an important way to regain some control over your health.

Why should you quit now? No matter how long you've been smoking, continued smoking is bad for your health in the short run by affecting your lungs, heart, and circulation. While you are receiving and recovering from cancer treatments, avoiding tobacco may make it easier for your *healthy* cells to recover. Although you may feel worse for a while after quitting because your body is used to the nicotine, your lungs, heart, and circulation will begin to experience the benefits almost immediately.

There are long-term benefits to quitting now, too. Even if you have smoked or chewed tobacco for many years, quitting now will increase your chance of avoiding certain problems that can occur months or years after your cancer treatments are over. In long-term survivors who continue to smoke, some problems can occur more often, earlier, or in more severe form. For example, compared to people who quit smoking after being diagnosed with cancer of the head or neck, people who continue smoking have an enormously higher risk of developing a second cancer of the head or neck even if they are cured of the first cancer. People who receive radiation to the chest have a much higher risk of developing lung cancer if they continue smoking than if they quit.

It is never too late to quit smoking or chewing tobacco. Use the threat of your cancer to help motivate you to quit for good.

What if I want to stop smoking but find quitting too stressful? Isn't it bad for my health to add on extra stress?

Many people who quit smoking feel awful for a while, which is stressful. Cancer is stressful enough, so you may want to avoid adding extra stress when given a choice. When you continue to smoke, you avoid the immediate discomforts of nicotine withdrawal, but you pay a great price. The chemical effects of tobacco *add* major stresses on your body because of the immediate and chronic changes they cause. In general, the health risks of continued smoking outweigh the risks associated with the stress of quitting.

If you enjoy tobacco, quitting will mean giving up something that gives you pleasure. You may feel sad and miss the good feelings you enjoyed while using tobacco. Like any sacrifice, you are doing it for a greater good: to maximize your chance of recovery. Remember that the discomforts of withdrawal are linked to a powerful step you are taking to help *improve your health*. There are many effective ways to help reduce the physical and emotional discomforts of quitting tobacco. Get help from experts if quitting is difficult for you.

Quitting tobacco is something positive you can do to help your recovery.

MEDICATION

What are my medicines?

Keep a written list of the names, amounts (dosages), and schedule of how you take your medications because:

- If you are tired, nervous, or groggy at the time of your visit, it will be easier for you and your doctor to review your medications.
- In an emergency situation, the doctors and nurses will need to know the names, amounts, and schedule of all your medications. A written list makes it easier for you or someone with you to provide this important information quickly.

- A written list that is shared with your doctors minimizes your chance of being given a medication that you should not get at this time. This is especially important when you see a number of doctors other than your oncologist, such as a cardiologist or gynecologist.
- A doctor treating you who is unfamiliar with your case can care for you more easily.

What medications should I include in my list?

All of them! Write down all prescription and nonprescription medicines, including over-the-counter medicines and alternative therapies. Include anything you are taking for:

- Cancer
- Pain
- Nausea or poor appetite
- Immune function
- Sleep
- Bowel function
- Depression
- Weight loss or gain
- All other medical conditions (stomach ulcers, infection, hormonal imbalance, and so on)
- Nutritional supplementation (vitamins, liquid diets, etc.)

Do I have to take all these prescribed medicines?

Your doctors will assume that you are taking all your prescribed medicines unless you tell them otherwise. Speak to your doctor before stopping or changing any medicines. There may be a significant danger to stopping a medicine without medical supervision; your doctors may need to change how often they see you or check a blood test.

When it comes to some medicines (e.g., some chemotherapy, some antibiotics, some pain medicines), it is critical that you take them exactly on time. If not taken exactly as directed, the medicines may not work or may cause problems. Other medicines do not demand such tight control. Find out how important it is to take each medicine on time.

Some medicines, so-called p.r.n. (*pro re nata*) medicines, are to be taken only as needed. "As needed" does not mean to wait until the symptom is unbearable; oftentimes the medicines work best when taken at the first sign of the problem. Some p.r.n. medicines can be taken as often as needed with no limit; other p.r.n. medicines should be taken only up to a maximum number of times a day. Make sure that you understand when and how to use each of your medicines, and the common side effects of each one.

How do I keep track of my medications?

You may be taking more pills than you normally take. Some cancer treatments require a complicated schedule of pill taking that changes from week to week, or month to month. Taking pills correctly is a big job when you are stressed or not feeling well.

One way to keep track of your medications is with a pill-minder. These handy plastic pillboxes are sold in pharmacies and grocery stores. Once a week, you fill them with your pills. If you take medication twice a day, it is best to get the pill-minder that has two slots for each day. For medication taken three times per day, get the pill-minder with three slots per day, and so on.

Seeing pills in your pill-minder will help remind you to take that dose. Pill-minders also provide excellent backup when you are not sure if you have taken a certain dose. As long as you are careful when you fill it with the week's medicines, during the week you can simply check your pill-minder whenever you want to make sure you took your medicine. Another advantage to pill-minders is that if the pharmacy accidentally gives you the wrong number of pills, you will discover the error when you fill your pill-minder. Otherwise, you might look in your pill bottle to take a dose on time, notice that there are too few or too many left, and then feel uncertain as to whether or not you took your dose properly.

Another way to keep track of your medicines is a medication list similar to that used in a hospital. Appendix D contains a sample list that you can copy or modify to fit your needs. Keep the week's list with your medications, and check off each dose as you take it. Pill-minders and medication lists will make the job easier and safer, and thus reduce your stress.

Taking your medicines correctly is an important job.

HAIR LOSS

Is hair loss expected?

Radiation can cause hair loss (**alopecia**) at the sites that have been radiated. Some chemotherapy causes hair loss. This is because the treatments work by damaging or killing all the rapidly dividing cells that they reach. Baldness is temporary in most cases, although high-dose radiation to the scalp can cause permanent hair loss. Hair loss due to chemotherapy affects all body hair, including eyebrows, eyelashes, axillary (armpit) hair, pubic hair, and the hair on your arms and legs. Your doctor or nurse can advise you as to the likelihood of hair loss or thinning based on experience with your particular treatments. No one can predict exactly how, if, or when you will lose your hair.

Being bald can be traumatic. It makes you look different than you did before, different than other people, and "like a cancer patient." Be reassured by your hair loss that the therapy is affecting dividing cells, including your cancer cells.

If I do not lose my hair, or my hair starts to grow back during therapy, is the therapy still working on my cancer?

Yes. There are people whose hair loss is minimal despite receiving medicines that usually cause total baldness. It is not uncommon to have hair start to grow back during therapy. These people have the same chance of improvement or recovery from their cancer as people who completely lose their hair.

When will I lose my hair?

If you lose your hair, it will probably be within a few weeks of your first or second round of treatment. Some people begin to lose hair a week after their first chemotherapy. How the hair comes out is variable. Your hair may gradually thin out over weeks, or it may fall out in clumps over one to two days. If you have long hair, it's a good idea to get a short, stylish haircut before or when you start to lose your hair because long hair that falls out can pull on the remaining long hair, causing clumps. Also, many patients find that it decreases the emotional trauma to go from short hair to no hair than from long hair to no hair.

Should I order a wig?

Maybe. If there is a high likelihood that you will lose your hair, and you think that you will want a wig, arranging to get a wig before you start losing your hair has some advantages:

- You can match your hair exactly.
- Your wig will be ready for use when you first start to lose hair (or will be ready soon, if custom-made).
- You will have time to practice with it and get it the way you like it before you really need to wear it.
- It may be easier to go to the wig salon before you start therapy.

There can be a couple of disadvantages to buying a wig right away. If you are now recovering from surgery or other medical problems, it may be easier to go to the wig salon later. After going through the trouble and expense of buying a wig, you may not lose as much hair as expected and you may not need it. Of course, you always can get fitted and then save the information (wig style, color, etc.) until after you are sure that you want to order a wig.

Bring one friend or family member with you when you choose your wig. This will make it easier to decide which wig is best, as well as help you to remember everything that you are told. You can find out about reputable wig salons from your oncologist, your nurse, other patients, or your local chapter of the American Cancer Society. There are important differences between fashion wigs and medical wigs, so specify that you need a medical wig.

Is a wig covered by my insurance policy?

Some cancer organizations make wigs available to patients as a free service. Wigs are covered by some insurance policies. Have your oncologist write a prescription for a "cranial prosthesis for alopecia secondary to chemotherapy (or radiation therapy)." Cranial prosthesis is the technical name for a medical wig. Ask your oncologist to avoid calling it a hair prosthesis or wig; insurance companies tend to be less enthusiastic about reimbursing when the prescription is phrased this way. File the prescription with the receipt from the wig salon.

PAIN CONTROL

What is causing my pain?

Pain is bodily distress, and can be caused by cancer and cancer therapy. This can occur because of:

- Cancer pressing on a nerve, organ, or vessel
- Recent surgery
- A broken bone due to cancer or surgery
- A blockage (such as of a blood vessel, digestive tube, or urinary tract)
- Skin or bowel changes from radiation
- Mouth irritation from chemotherapy
- Infection
- Swelling

The degree of your pain is influenced by nonphysical factors such as:

- Your anxiety and fear
- The meaning of your pain to you
- Your sense of control over your pain
- Your patterns of response to pain

If my pain is getting worse, is my cancer growing?

Not necessarily. Although worsening pain can be caused by cancer that is growing, many *other* problems can cause new or increased pain even as the cancer responds well to treatment. If your pain is worse, yet all objective indicators say that your cancer is improving, the pain is probably *not* due to progressive cancer.

How does anxiety affect pain?

Anxiety and pain feed each other in a vicious cycle. Pain can cause you to feel anxious; anxiety can increase your perception of pain. Both are treatable symptoms. If you are at all anxious about your pain (and most people are), get attention for both your pain *and* your anxiety. For more about the treatment of anxiety, see page 170.

What other factors affect pain?

Depending on the source of your pain, the quality and degree of pain may be affected by certain activities, weather conditions, fatigue or sleep deprivation, depression, malnutrition, or bowel or bladder function. For example, constipation may worsen pelvic discomfort. Fatigue lowers your threshold for pain. Attention to these elements may help alleviate your pain even when the cause cannot be corrected.

Do I have to tell my health-care team about my pain?

Yes. Yes. Yes. Cancer pain is very treatable. Sometimes referred to as "the fourth vital sign" (along with temperature, blood pressure, and pulse), pain is your body's way of telling you and your health-care team that something is wrong. When you report any new pain or change in your pain, your doctors and nurses can check for a problem or complication that may be easy to treat now and much harder to take care of later. The other reason to tell your doctors and nurses about any new or persistent pain is *to get you relief* while the cause for your pain is being determined.

Some people have the mistaken notion that pain is part of cancer, so they just accept it. For others, it is socially unacceptable to complain about pain. Being a patient is not a social situation, and *reporting pain to your doctors is not complaining.* Controlling pain is a team effort. Your doctors want to hear about any discomforts you are having so that appropriate evaluation and treatment can be done in a timely manner. Don't assume that your doctor knows you are hurting. Pain will not show up on your blood tests or scans; you have to tell your doctors and nurses.

Your pain is unique. Optimum pain management for you is unique.

What should I tell my doctor about my pain?

Before you call or see your doctor, prepare the answers to the following questions:

- When did the pain first start, or begin to get worse?
- Where is the pain? (Include all areas involved.)
- How severe is the pain? (See next question.)
- What kind of pain is it? Is it sharp like a knife, dull like a toothache, burning, cramping, or like an electric shock?
- Is the pain constant, or does it come and go (or wax and wane)?
- Is there any numbness or tingling?
- What have you done to relieve the pain? How much relief have you gotten, and how long does this relief last?
- Have you ever had pain like this before? What was it caused by in the past? What helped relieve the pain in the past?

How do I describe the severity of my pain?

Your doctors and family need to have some idea of the severity of your pain if they are to help you. One way to communicate the severity of your pain is to rate the pain, where 0 = no pain, 5 = moderate pain, and 10 = the worst pain ever. Rating the pain not only gives some idea of your current level of pain; it also offers a way to measure the change in your pain over time and with treatment.

Another approach is to compare it to other pain you've had: "The stomach cramps feel like when I had a minor stomach virus" or "almost as bad as when I was in labor." "My leg hurts like when I've bumped it against a table" or "like when I broke it a few years ago."

Others will have a clearer idea of the severity of your pain if you describe how the pain is interfering with your daily activities. For example, does the pain make it difficult to walk, get dressed,

sit at a desk, lift a gallon of milk, and so on? Does the pain interfere with your sleep? Is the pain making you afraid or depressed?

How is pain controlled?

Doctors usually start with the mildest therapies and gradually
work up to stronger therapies until pain control is achieved.
Almost all cancer pain can be treated with pills (if you can swallow and your digestive tract is working).

Mild pain is usually first treated with non-narcotics (nonopi-
ates) such as:

- **Analgesics** (pain relievers) like Tylenol®
- Nonsteroidal anti-inflammatory medicines like aspirin or
  ibuprofen (e.g., Motrin® or Advil®)

These medicines have a limit, called the ceiling, above which you
get no better pain relief, but you will see increased risks and side
effects.

Moderate pain or mild pain that does not respond to
non-narcotics is treated with pain relievers called weak **opioids**
or narcotic analgesics. Examples include codeine, Darvon®,
Darvocet®, Tylox®, Percocet®, and Percodan®. The dose of
these medicines does not have a ceiling and, *with proper supervision by a doctor*, a dose usually can be found that will relieve pain.
Oftentimes, non-narcotics are used along with narcotics.

Severe pain or milder pain that does not respond to non-
narcotics and weak opioids usually will respond to strong opioids
such as morphine (a short-acting medicine) and fentanyl patches
or methadone pills (longer-acting medicines).

Adjuvants are medicines that usually are prescribed for non-
pain medical problems but that also offer some benefit in the
treatment of pain. They can play an important role in the treatment of mild, moderate, and severe pain. Examples include
antidepressants, antinausea medicines, antianxiety medicines,
anticonvulsants, antispasmotics, and stimulants. Other measures used in the treatment of cancer pain include radiation
therapy and steroids.

Be sure your doctors know all the medicines you are taking (prescription and over-the-counter) and all your drug allergies before they prescribe pain medicines for you.

How is pain medicine taken?

Most pain medications are taken orally in pill or liquid form. This is the preferred route when you are able to swallow and digest food. Pain medicines also can be taken

- Rectally—a suppository dissolves in the rectum and is absorbed by the body; useful when vomiting is a problem
- Transdermally—a gel or medicine-impregnated patch is placed on the skin
- Intranasally—a liquid is sprayed into the nose
- By injection
     Subcutaneously—just under the skin using a small needle
     Intravenously— in the vein through an intravenous line
     Intrathecally—into the spinal fluid
     Subdermally or intramuscularly—deep under the skin or
        in a muscle

If one mild pain medicine doesn't work, does that mean I need stronger medicines?

Not necessarily. Many people do not get good relief with one type of mild medicine but get excellent relief with another. Or, you may not get good relief with a low dose of one medicine but may get good relief with a higher dose or a combination of two different mild pain relievers. Nobody can predict which particular medicines or combination of medicines will work well for your pain. That's why it is so important to work with your physicians as a team to find the optimum medications for you.

If my doctor prescribed morphine, does that mean I am dying?

No. Morphine is not reserved for dying patients. Morphine is a safe and effective pain reliever when prescribed by someone experienced in the treatment of cancer pain. It is used often to control pain during early phases of the disease, enabling many to resume their usual activities at work and home.

When do I need to call my doctors about my pain?

Now, if your pain is severe. Call your doctors' office if your pain is

- keeping you from getting up or walking;
- causing you to have a poor appetite or difficulty eating;
- interfering with your sleep;
- causing you to be upset, afraid, or depressed;
- not controlled at all times with the prescribed treatment;
- controlled but now you have a new pain; or
- now associated with numbness, tingling, or burning sensations.

How long should it take a dose of pain medication to work?

In general, you should get some pain relief within fifteen to thirty minutes of a shot, within an hour of taking oral medication, and within six hours of placing a patch. It may take a day or two to get your pain under control with a regimen that ultimately proves successful. Many factors affect how quickly you'll experience relief and how long your relief will last. Find out what to expect. Let your health-care team know if it is taking a long time to get relief, the relief is incomplete, or your pain is returning long before it's time to take another dose of medication.

What is breakthrough pain?

Pain that occurs between scheduled doses of medication is called **breakthrough pain**. If breakthrough pain occurs infrequently, your physician will prescribe a "rescue dose" of medication, so named because it rescues or saves you from pain until your next dose is due. If breakthrough pain occurs often, your routine pain medications probably need adjusting.

Can my pain medicines cause side effects?

Yes. Pain medicines, like all medicines, can cause their own problems. Certain side effects are common, such as:

- Constipation
- Dry mouth and nasal passages (nose and sinuses)
- Nausea
- Drowsiness, clouded thinking

Ask your nurses and doctors about anticipated side effects and measures you can take to prevent them. For example, the constipating effect of narcotic medicines can be minimized by drinking enough fluids, taking stool softeners, eating high-fiber foods, and avoiding constipating foods such as cheese or chocolate. Ask your doctor what measures you can take safely. Don't delay in letting your doctors know if you are having side effects. Most problems that require treatment are more easily managed if addressed early. Your doctors will let you know if you can expect a particular side effect to decrease or resolve on its own after a few days or weeks as your body gets used to the medicines.

Many people refuse pain medicines because they want to be as alert as possible. It's important to realize that *uncontrolled pain* can lead to fatigue and confusion, too. By giving you relief of your pain, effective medicines can lead to an overall increase in your energy and clearheadedness.

Optimum therapy gives you good pain control with minimum side effects.

What is a drug reaction?

A drug reaction is not the same as a side effect, because it usually is more serious and often results in a change in therapy. If you are allergic to a pain medicine or the medicine is too strong for you, you need to call your doctor or nurse *immediately*. Any of the following symptoms can signal a drug reaction:

- Skin rash, itching, or swelling of the face
- Confusion
- Sleepiness so that someone else has great difficulty waking you
- Nausea or vomiting without relief
- Being unable to urinate

- Being unable to hold in urine or stool (a new problem)
- Severe trembling, uncontrolled muscle movements, or seizures (convulsions or "fits")
- Hallucinations
- Ringing in the ears

Drug reactions are not common. Some drug reactions can be reversed with medical treatment. All drug reactions need to be brought to the attention of your doctors and nurses. When in doubt about a symptom, call the office.

Are there ways to relieve pain without medicines?

Yes. Various nonpharmacologic measures also can help relieve your pain. Ask your doctors and nurses about measures, such as:

- Taking warm showers, or applying warm water bottles to painful areas. Do not place on skin that has received any radiation in the past two months or so, or on skin that is irritated or broken!
- Applying cool cloths or ice packs to painful areas
- Menthol-containing creams and lotions
- Massage
- Biofeedback; hypnosis
- TENS (transcutaneous electrical nerve stimulation)
- Acupuncture

Other measures such as avoiding painful activities, positioning painful areas with pillows, distraction, self-relaxation, and humor may help take the edge off, too.

What if I'm afraid of having uncontrolled pain?

Remember the facts: Safe and effective measures can control pain. Eighty-five percent of patients with cancer pain obtain relief with pain pills alone. For almost all the 15 percent of people for whom pills are not enough, there are effective therapies that provide excellent pain control. Difficult-to-control pain may indicate the need for referral to one of the many pain-control physicians. These specialists work with your regular doctors to help alleviate your pain when the usual measures do not offer adequate relief. Sometimes it takes a trial of a few different approaches before optimum pain control is achieved, but you can expect to get good pain relief. Pain can be controlled best through a team effort with your doctors. Let your doctors know if you have pain or if the pain medicine is causing another problem.

You have a right to good pain control.

What if my pain is not improving?

It may take awhile to get your pain well controlled because pain medicines take time to build up in the bloodstream. Also, finding the best dose for you can take time: Doctors often start out prescribing milder pain medicines because it is easier to add more medicine than to deal with a drug reaction from receiving more medicine than you need. Keep working with your doctors on your pain until your pain is well controlled.

Keep your doctors informed of any persistent pain.

Should I be worried about becoming addicted to the pain medicine?

No. Medicine that is used properly to control pain rarely leads to drug addiction. You will be able to stop using the medicines as soon as your pain is under control. Note that *physical dependence* (the need to taper off drugs to avoid withdrawal symptoms) and **tolerance** (the need for higher doses of medication to get the same pain control) are not the same as *addiction* (wanting the medicine for anything other than control of pain).

Don't suffer needless pain out of fear of becoming addicted to effective pain medications. Along the same lines, don't worry about exhausting your options for pain control and having nothing left to use if you develop more severe pain later. We now know that this concern is unfounded and only deprives you of effective measures that can offer relief from mild or moderate pain you're having now. Taking pain medication regularly may control your pain more effectively because you sustain a necessary blood level of the medication. *Don't tough it out.*

What if I have (or had in the past) a problem with or addiction to drugs or alcohol?

Let your doctors know if addiction has ever been a problem for you. Drug addiction, like diabetes or heart disease, is a medical problem. Your physicians' full knowledge of your history of addiction helps to

- avoid potential complications with the cancer treatments that are related to prior drug or alcohol addiction;
- avoid new problems with drug or alcohol addiction;
- optimize your pain control.

When administered under proper supervision, medications can be prescribed that will provide good pain relief without stirring up serious problems with addiction. On the one hand, don't deny yourself adequate pain medication for fear of causing uncontrolled addiction—an understandable fear if you've over-come bad times due to drugs or alcohol. On the other hand, if you feel that your doctors are reluctant to prescribe adequate pain medication for fear of triggering an addiction problem, ask for referral to a pain specialist who can provide guidance for this special circumstance.

What if my insurance company says they won't pay for my pain medication?

Good pain managament is a vital part of good cancer care. You have a right to available methods of pain control. Many resources are available to help patients who are uninsured or whose insurance companies do not cover the complete costs of pain mangagment. Some good starting points are:

- Your health-care team. They may be able to connect you with patient advocates and health-care agencies in your local community who can help you find funding for pain medications.
- The American Cancer Society. Your state division may have funds to assist in the payment of pain medications.

- The National Coalition for Cancer Survivorship (see Appendix C)
- The Patient Advocate Foundation (PAF)
                753 Thimble Shoals Blvd., Suite B
                Newport News, VA 23606
                Phone: 800-532-5274
                Fax: 757-873-8999 780
                www.patientadvocate.org

What if my family and I disagree about how much pain medicine I should be taking?

Only you know how much pain you have, how much it is bothering you, and how well you are tolerating the pain medicines. Everyone has a different pain threshold, and everyone handles pain medicine in a unique way. If you feel that you are getting good pain relief, let your family know this. If they still feel that you are undermedicated, discuss with them why they feel this way. Your nurse and doctor can help you and your family understand how to optimize your pain control. You are the one in charge of your pain control.

You don't earn any brownie points for enduring pain!

NUTRITION

Should I be on a special diet?

Yes. Good nutrition is an important part of your care and will contribute to your sense of well-being. Nourishment is needed for:

- daily functioning (breathing, moving, and so on);
- repair of injured or damaged tissues;
- fighting cancer;
- fighting infection;
- dealing with the bodily changes due to cancer therapy.

Most people who have cancer or are receiving cancer treatment have an increased need for calories, protein, and fluids. Your situation may require special nutritional supplements or dietary restrictions. You can ask for specific guidance from your doctor or nurse. A nutritionist may be involved in your assessment and follow-up.

Why do many people lose weight during treatment for cancer?

Approximately half of the people with cancer have unintended weight loss due to cancer-induced changes in their bodies. Some cancers and/or cancer therapies are associated with one or more of the following:

- Decreased appetite and/or taste appreciation
- Nausea and/or vomiting
- Trouble swallowing
- Diarrhea
- Muscle breakdown
- Poor absorption of nutrients from food
- Inefficient use of absorbed nutrients
- Decreased fat storage
- Fasting (not eating, in preparation for tests or surgery)

What can I do to avoid weight loss?

If you are able to eat but have a poor appetite:

- Think of eating as part of your treatment, and something you can do to help yourself get well and feel better.
- Eat what you can eat within any dietary restrictions advised. Don't worry about eating "breakfast foods" at breakfast time, and so on. If you find a few items that appeal to you, eat them as often as you like. Yet, try to vary your foods as much as possible to avoid getting burned out on any particular foods.
- Eat when you can eat, preferably small meals and nutritious snacks throughout the day.
- If food tastes metallic, try using plastic utensils.
- Discuss food preparation with your nurse or dietician.

If you have difficulty eating solids, try liquid supplements in addition to or in place of meals. Supplements go down fast and easy, and you will be nourishing yourself almost as if you were eating solid food. These can be bought without a prescription from pharmacies and some grocery stores. Ask your doctor if you should use a liquid supplement that has fiber in it. If you are unable to eat, your doctor may discuss the possibility of starting tube feedings (liquid feedings through a tube placed into your digestive tract) or intravenous feedings called **total parenteral nutrition (TPN)**.

If I was on a special diet at the time of my diagnosis, should I continue it?

Maybe. If you are on a diabetic, low-cholesterol, high-calcium, lactose-free, low-calorie, or other special diet, discuss with your doctor whether any changes need to be made. During treatment, your need for the dietary restrictions may be increased or decreased. Some special diets may interfere with your cancer therapy.

What about the recommendations to eat a low-fat diet to prevent cancer and heart disease?

Recommendations about diet from the American Cancer Society and the American Heart Association are intended for healthy people who are trying to prevent the development of cancer and heart disease. The balance of risks and benefits may be different when your body is dealing with cancer treatment. Right now your top dietary priority is providing the nutrients needed to fight cancer and recover from treatments. You can worry about preventing future disease after you have completed treatment and recovery.

Why does my diet seem to be the focus of my family's attention?

Concern over your diet may cause strain among family members. You may disagree with them about what to eat, when to eat, or how well you are eating. For many families, cancer and its treatment are new and difficult to understand. Your diet is something with which family members feel familiar and comfortable. Since your diet is important to your well-being, it may provide a concrete way that they can participate in your care. Food is also an important means by which loved ones show affection. Concern with your diet and attempts to serve special foods are ways that family members may express their love for you.

Share with your doctor or nurse your family's concerns, preferably with family members present. Clarify your dietary needs and whether your current diet is optimal. Tell your family exactly how involved you want them to be in your food selection and preparation. Let family members know if you appreciate their involvement for both the assistance and comfort it provides, or if you see their input as yet one further loss of independence or threat to your sense of self.

Do people ever gain weight while being treated for cancer?

Yes, many people gain weight during therapy for cancer. This can be due to decreased physical activity and/or to medication such as steroids. When your cancer is associated with swelling or fluid accumulation, you can gain weight without adding any fat. You may even be *losing* muscle mass and fat despite apparent weight gain. If you have been overweight for a long time, it may be very disappointing to gain additional weight, especially if you were expecting easy weight loss to be a welcomed side effect of having cancer. Even if you have never had a weight problem, weight gain can be distressing. You can avoid some weight gain by limiting your consumption of "empty" calories (snack chips, cookies, and candy). Staying as active as your medical condition allows will also help (see page 121).

If I am overweight, can I try to lose weight?

In most cases, this is not a good time to try to lose weight. Weight loss due to cancer or poor intake of food is not a healthy weight loss. Dieting may deprive your body of the fuel it needs to clear the cancer cells or recover from the treatments. You can decide to do something about your weight when you are done with treatment and recovery.

If excessive weight is contributing to your medical problems, your doctor may recommend a weight-loss diet that also provides the nutrients needed to optimize your response to treatments.

Is there a special diet to prevent cancer?

The American Cancer Society makes these recommendations:

• Avoid obesity.
• Eat a low-fat diet.

- Include fiber in your diet.
- Eat cruciferous vegetables (cabbage, broccoli, Brussels sprouts, cauliflower).
- Eat four to six helpings of fruits and vegetables daily.
- Avoid excessive alcohol consumption.
- Be moderate in your consumption of salt-cured, smoked, and nitrite-cured foods.

What about all the stories of people being cured with a macrobiotic (or other) diet?

Most people with terminal cancer who follow a macrobiotic (grain and vegetable) or other unconventional diet as their only treatment are not cured of their cancer. You may find well-documented stories of people with terminal cancer going into remission or being cured after adhering to a special diet, but many of these people also received conventional therapies so you can't know what role their diet played in their recoveries. For those exceptional individuals who recovered without any conventional therapies, diet may indeed have been a factor, if not the main reason, for the remarkable recovery. However, anecdotes are not scientific study, and you have no way to know if such a diet is useful in the treatment of cancer.

A macrobiotic diet is not appetizing to many people. Trying to keep to it could be stressful or discouraging—not a state of mind conducive to healing. Unusual diets may not provide the necessary nutrients needed by your body at this time.

Your diet is one essential element of healing that is under your control. Choose and follow a diet that will provide the fuel and nutrients needed to give you the best overall chance of getting well and staying well.

EXERCISE

Why is exercise important during cancer therapy?

Numerous studies have shown that *moderate-intensity* exercise decreases stress and improves the quality of life of patients during and after cancer therapy. Also, moderate-intensity exercise improves certain measures of immune function. Researchers expect the current studies being done on cancer patients to confirm what already has been shown in patients with other diseases such as heart disease and diabetes: Fitness is associated with improved outcome and decreased mortality.

What are the benefits of exercising during cancer treatment?

Studies on cancer survivors have demonstrated many physical benefits, including:

- increased energy and endurance;
- decreased nausea; improved appetite;
- decreased muscle wasting; increased strength, mobility, range of motion;
- decreased complications from surgery;
- improved blood flow to limbs, which may decrease blood clots;
- improved red-blood-cell production, which can help the heart and lungs;
- improved sleep;
- prevention of weight gain during treatments that often cause weight gain.

Emotional benefits include:

- decreased stress, depression, and anxiety;
- increased independence (related to improved strength and mobility);
- improved self-esteem, pride, confidence;
- increased opportunities for social interactions related to being more fit;
- increased sense of control.

If you were involved in an exercise program before your diagnosis, you probably will find it fairly easy to continue your program with modifications as needed. Many survivors report a sense of relief and hopefulness when exercising because they are doing something that feels "normal."

What are the downsides of exercising during cancer therapy?

Although moderate-intensity exercise shows benefits, *intense* exercise such as running a marathon has been associated with suppression of the immune system. For this reason, the usual recommendation is to avoid high-intensity sports and exercises during cancer treatment even if you did them regularly before your diagnosis. Depending on your choice of exercise, you could suffer an injury that might complicate your recovery. If you push too hard or ignore warning signs of problems, you may feel worse instead of better.

Properly supervised exercise is a low-risk, high-gain endeavor.

What kind of exercises should I do?

A good exercise program is safe, enjoyable, and effective in helping maximize your strength, endurance, flexibility, and level of functioning. Studies are under way to answer the question of what constitutes the optimal type, frequency, duration, and intensity of exercise during cancer therapy. Make sure that your exercise program

- is approved of by your oncologist;
- is tailored to your physical condition;
- includes warm-up and cool-down periods;
- includes exercises that help strength, flexibility, and cardiovascular conditioning;
- builds up over time to moderate intensity for thirty to sixty minutes every day;
- is flexible to allow for fluctuations in your condition;
- is fun.

Walking is the most popular activity and the one studied most in research on exercise in cancer survivors. Brisk walking doesn't require special training or equipment, although you need to wear good shoes. If fitness walking for thirty to sixty minutes in one session is not possible, you can integrate three to six ten-minute brisk walks into your daily routine and get similar benefit. Cycling is another popular exercise for cancer survivors. Being seated helps when you have catheters, lymphedema, significant anemia, or difficulty with standing, weight bearing, or balance. The buoyancy of water makes exercises done in water the preferred approach for certain patients with muscle or joint problems. Alternative exercise and stretching methods include yoga, tai chi, and qigong.

Any activity that gets your heart rate up for a sustained period of time and that builds strength and flexibility is good. Hiking, dancing, gardening, sports, and even washing your car and playing tag with your grandchildren can improve your level of fitness.

Are there any special precautions I should take?

During cancer treatment, your body is subjected to many stresses and may be weakened in certain ways. If you have

- a low red-blood-cell count (i.e., you are anemic), you may need to decrease the intensity of your workout;
- a low white-blood-cell count, you may need to avoid infection-prone environments and equipment. Swimming in pools or lakes may be discouraged;
- a low platelet count or are taking blood-thinning medications, you may need to avoid high-impact exercise. Avoid activities that could result in cuts or falls that would predispose you to bleeding;
- had vomiting and/or diarrhea, you may need to have the electrolytes in your blood checked to be sure that your sodium and potassium levels are adequate for safe exercise;
- lung disease or are receiving treatments that affect the lungs (such as certain chemotherapy agents or chest irradiation), you may need to decrease the intensity of your workout, especially if you get short of breath;
- bone disease such as metastases in your bones, you may need to avoid high-impact exercises or the use of excessive weights that could trigger a bone fracture;
- lymphedema (see page 130), you need to avoid activities that might exacerbate the swelling;
- difficulty with balance or coordination, or sensation, you may need to avoid activities such as walking on uneven ground that could result in injury;

• a fever, you should hold off on your exercises until the fever resolves or your doctor has evaluated you and feels it is okay to exercise with fever.

An exercise program can be designed that will accommodate almost any restrictions due to your condition. Even if you are very sick, exercises can be done in a chair or in bed to improve your overall fitness and make an important difference in your quality of life.

What if my oncologist never discusses exercise?

If your oncologist doesn't bring it up first, ask him or her to

• prescribe an exercise program, or review a program that you would like to do;
• outline any special precautions you need to take;
• advise you on any signs or symptoms for which you should stop exercising.

If your oncologist or general practitioner does not feel comfortable advising you about exercise, find out if any cancer rehabilitation services are available through one of your local hospitals, support groups, wellness centers, or athletic centers such as the YMCA. Some exercise physiotherapists, sports trainers, and physical therapists have special training in the care of cancer survivors, but a physician's prescription is advisable and often necessary.

Should I ever stop exercising?

Yes. Stop exercising and call your doctor right away if you develop any of the following during or after exercise:

• Pain, bleeding, swelling
• Dizziness or increased weakness
• Blurred vision or headache
• Chest pain or palpitations
• Numbness or tingling
• Shortness of breath that doesn't resolve quickly
• New symptom

If you are feeling poorly after one of your treatments, or you are running a fever or have developed a new symptom, you probably need to stop exercising for a day or two until the problem resolves or you and your physician know what's going on. Your physician can let you know when it is safe to resume exercise.

What if I feel like I don't have the time or energy to exercise while dealing with the demands of treatment?

Think about why you are going through your cancer treatments: to regain your health. Fitness is an essential element of good health. Getting daily exercise is one important way to help improve your sense of well-being during treatment and to speed your recovery after completion of treatment.

What if I'm having trouble getting started?

If you don't feel motivated, or you were sedentary before your diagnosis, try

- setting short-term goals that are achievable;
- slowly building up your exercise intensity and duration;
- finding an exercise partner;
- charting and rewarding your progress;
- adding variety;
- setting long-term goals.

You may need to start with one to two minutes of very light exercise per session, and build up over weeks or months until you can do moderate intensity for thirty to sixty minutes per day (or less, if that is the maximum you can do). Every little bit helps. Keep your ultimate goal in mind: feeling better and getting better.

Exercise is an important element of a healing program that is under your control.

FATIGUE

What if I'm very tired?

Fatigue is a very common problem in cancer patients. Progress in cancer care has led to improved treatments that prevent or relieve more dramatic symptoms such as vomiting and pain. Consequently, fatigue is now receiving more attention from patients, nurses, and doctors.

Fatigue is defined as a feeling of weariness during or following exertion, but may be experienced as any combination of:

- Feeling tired
- Lack of energy or stamina
- Difficulty staying awake
- Difficulty concentrating or learning new information
- Irritability or emotional lability (ever-changing emotions, such as crying spells or bursts of anger)
- Loss of interest in people or things around you

Why am I so tired?

Any of the following possible causes may contribute to your fatigue over the course of your treatments:

- Your cancer
- Medications such as chemotherapy, interferons, pain medicines, antiseizure medicines
- **Anemia** (low red-blood-cell counts)
- Chemical imbalance(s) such as low potassium
- Hormonal changes
- The physical drain from your body's efforts to heal
- Breathing difficulties
- Changes in your nervous system caused by your disease or treatments
- Infection
- Emotional factors such as anxiety, depression, frustration, boredom, or conflict

- Malnutrition
- Change in sleep pattern
- Deconditioning (getting out of shape from lack of activity)
- Overexertion
- Consumption of alcohol, caffeine, nicotine

Usually, fatigue is cumulative and gets progressively worse as treatment continues. However, your energy may improve if the fatigue caused by your treatments is overshadowed by the improvement in energy associated with getting rid of the cancer and correcting problems such as anemia or chemical imbalances. Over the next few months, the specific cause(s) of your fatigue may change even if the level of your fatigue stays the same.

What if I am more tired than other patients?

How you feel is how you feel. Your specific circumstances are unique before and during treatment, as are the reactions of your mind and body to everything. Comparing your energy level with someone else's doesn't help anyone. Try to focus on how you can feel as well as possible in the short run, while maximizing your chances for a smooth and complete recovery.

What if my energy fluctuates?

Many patients note wide fluctuations in their energy level from week to week, day to day, and even hour to hour. After awhile, you may be able to detect a pattern to your vigor. So many factors affect energy that predictions may not be reliable, if they can be made at all. This variation is expected.

Can I do anything to improve my energy?

Some level of fatigue may be an unavoidable side effect of your illness. Your doctors and nurses can help you take the following steps to minimize your tiredness:

- Eat nourishing meals and snacks.
- Adjust your medications whenever possible (for example, your doctor may be able to prescribe different pain medicines that give you equal pain relief but less sleepiness).

- Get attention for any anxiety, depression, anger.
- Include doctor-approved exercise in your daily routine (see page 123).
- Create a routine that includes adequate amounts of rest.
- Ensure that the quality of your sleep is good.
- Adjust your energy demands to meet your current limitations. You may need help learning how to do this.

What if I still feel tired despite getting a good night's sleep?

Don't be discouraged if you tire easily or you never feel refreshed no matter how much sleep you get. Cancer and most treatments can cause fatigue that persists despite adequate rest. However, sleeping well at night and taking a nap or two during the day may improve your energy significantly. As long as you are also getting enough daily physician-approved exercise and physical activity, good-quality rest recharges your body's batteries and may improve and speed your recovery. Let your doctors know if you can't relax or sleep well.

Slowing down can be frustrating, especially when you feel that your time is limited, but rest is a critical ingredient during treatment. Even while you are sitting still, treatments cause your body to work overtime, killing cancer cells and repairing normal cells.

Sleeping is not wasting time.

Am I hurting myself if I overexert myself?

Probably, especially if you don't get the rest your body needs. Most physical discomforts are signals that you need to change something that you are doing. For instance, when you break your leg, the pain discourages you from walking on it. If you ignore the signal and try to walk, you risk further injury. Feeling exhausted, achy, or irritable is the result of imbalances in your body or depleted energy stores. Fatigue, like pain, is your body's signal that it needs you to do something. In this case, you need rest. Pushing yourself when you are tired not only makes you feel worse; doing so may also deny your body the rest it needs to heal and deal with all the added stresses.

Can I get too much rest?

Yes. An attempt to save your energy by resting all the time can backfire and make you feel increasingly tired. Too much rest, especially bed rest, leads to deconditioning. Also, too many naps can make it difficult to get a good night's sleep, which creates a vicious cycle of daytime sleepiness and nighttime insomnia.

Try to maintain (or improve) your physical strength and condition. See if taking some of your daytime rests sitting up instead of lying flat in bed helps your energy. Your need for rest will fluctuate depending on what treatments you are receiving at the time, and the other physical and emotional stresses in your life. Talk with your doctors and nurses about how to get enough rest but not too much.

LYMPHEDEMA

What is lymphedema?

Lymphedema is swelling due to blockage of the lymphatic vessels. It is most often due to surgery or radiation therapy that damages these vessels. Although it can occur anywhere in the body, lymphedema is most noticeable and problematic when it affects the arm(s) or leg(s). Not only is the swelling unsightly, even disfiguring, if severe, it can be associated with pain, decreased range of motion of the affected limb, skin changes (hardening, thickening, breakdown), increased risk of serious infections of the nearby skin, and psychological distress.

Am I at risk of developing lymphedema?

You are at risk of developing lymphedema if you had

- surgery to remove lymph nodes from your axilla (armpit), inguinal region (groin), or pelvis;
- radiation to your axilla or inguinal region;
- damage to the larger lymph vessels from surgery or radiation;
- blood clots in your legs or pelvis.

Patients with melanoma, lymphoma, breast, prostate, testicular, bladder, gynecological, or other cancers often are at risk when their disease and/or treatment caused lymphatic damage. In general, your risk of developing lymphedema increases when

- many lymph nodes are removed from one area;
- infection or scarring of lymphatic tissue developes after surgery or radiation;
- you have both surgery and radiation to the same lymph node area.

What can I do to prevent lymphedema?

Prevention is the key and is best started immediately. If you are at risk yet haven't shown signs of this problem, don't be lulled into a false sense of security. Lymphedema can first appear weeks, months, years, or even decades after completion of successful treatment. From now on:

- Protect your limb(s) from any injuries or infections: Avoid having blood drawn or injections given into your affected limb; shave only with an electric razor; avoid cutting your cuticles; avoid insect bites and stings; avoid rapid changes in temperature associated with the use of ice packs or heating pads; avoid carrying a heavy bag on the affected arm; and so on.
- Minimize swelling: Elevate the affected limb; avoid constricting jewelry or elastic bands; avoid obesity.
- Prevent and treat infections: Keep the skin clean and moist; avoid sunburn; check skin for breakdown or signs of infection; wear long gloves when doing work that may result in scrapes, scratches, punctures, or burns; use a thimble when handling a needle or other sharp object; and so on.

Talk with your health-care team about special precautions you should take before traveling on an airplane, especially for long flights.

Call your doctor *immediately* if you develop increased heat or swelling in the limb, redness or a red streak, pain, fever, or chills.

What if I've developed some lymphedema already?

Lymphedema is treatable. Get specialized attention for your lymphedem as soon as possible. Some of the measures that may be recommended include:

- Elevating the limb periodically throughout the day
- Wearing a professionally fitted compression sleeve after treatment with a special pump or manual massage designed to help relieve lymphedema
- Beginning or continuing a doctor-approved exercise program

Be sure that any therapy is prescribed and administered by a medical professional trained in the treatment of lymphedema. Find out more about the prevention and treatment of lymphedema, as well as local services for treatment and support, from the National Lymphedema Network (800-541-3259; www.lymphnet.org).

WORK AND SCHOOL

Will I be able to continue working or going to school while I undergo testing?

A brief leave from work or school may be needed for:

- Recuperation from surgery or procedures
- Completion of your evaluation
- Emotional adjustment to your diagnosis
- Beginning treatment

Your medical situation may leave you little choice but to take at least a short leave of absence. Even if you feel well physically, adjusting to a diagnosis of cancer is a major stress that can make it difficult or impossible to do your job satisfactorily.

Some patients are able to continue their usual jobs. In fact, they find the routine and distraction of work comforting as the shock of the diagnosis wears off and reality sinks in. Many other people do better if they focus first on family matters, doctors' appointments and second opinions, insurance concerns, and getting a wig. Even when they are physically able to work, these people find that taking off a few days or weeks up-front is prudent because doing so allows them to get things in order and avoid a lot of little absences from work. Keep in mind that a long treatment regimen is like a marathon: If you sprint through the first few miles and try to take care of everything at work and home while dealing with your diagnosis and evaluation, you'll have less energy to cope with treatment later on.

Will I be able to continue working or studying while I undergo treatment?

Many people work or study full-time or part-time during cancer therapy. Whether you can work or continue school will depend on:

- How rigorous your treatment is
- How demanding your treatment schedule is
- How flexible your job or school is regarding schedules
- How physically and emotionally demanding your job or schoolwork is
- How well you are doing physically
- How well you are doing emotionally

Long-term leave may be needed if

- Treatment makes it difficult or impossible to perform your usual duties.
- Your work puts you at risk during treatment (for example, a pediatric nurse would be at risk of serious infection while undergoing some chemotherapy treatments).

Discuss with your doctor and your family how you should handle your immediate work or school situation.

Should I tell my boss, colleagues, coworkers, subordinates, students, or others about my cancer diagnosis?

How much you tell others will depend on your particular work relationships and circumstances, your health status, and your personality. The advantages of sharing your news are:

- You avoid misunderstandings about why you look or act differently than usual. Note that speculation can be worse than the truth.
- You will not have to put up as convincing a front on difficult days.
- You will not have to create excuses or explanations when you need to make schedule changes or if people notice any changes in you. Note that explaining yourself can be draining.
- You may find an important support system at work.

The disadvantages of sharing your news are:

- You may have to deal with other people's fears, concerns, and prejudices about your illness.
- You may have to deal with people's sympathetic concern for you ("How are you doing today?" "When is your next checkup?") on days when you feel great and would like to forget about cancer.
- You may be disappointed by some people's lack of concern or lack of sympathy when you need it.
- Well-meaning people may say things that are hurtful or stupid.

All states provide legal protection from discrimination due to a handicap. Much attention has been focused on the rights of cancer patients, and whether having cancer or having a history of cancer makes a person handicapped. An individual's legal protection in this regard varies from state to state.

GETTING HELP

Why should I ask for help?

You are dealing with the demands of your evaluation and treatment. You may be feeling any combination of physical, emotional, spiritual, and financial stress. If you seek and accept help, you can

- devote your time and energy to taking care of your medical needs, and the decisions ahead of you;

- have more time and energy to communicate with your family and friends, create a support network, and work through some of your feelings;
- get more rest.

Family and friends want to make things better for you. The only way they can help is by doing errands, making meals, talking, and listening. By asking others for help, you offer *them* an opportunity to enrich *their* lives.

In most cases, it is unrealistic and unfair to expect a spouse or life partner to provide all the help you need, even when he or she seems to want to do it all. The emotional and physical demands of your illness can take a severe toll on them after awhile. Getting assistance helps to prevent caregiver burnout.

Help yourself and help others by accepting help.

What kind of help do I need?

You may need help with:

- Meals
- Transportation to and from appointments
- Baby-sitting
- Transporting children to school, activities, or doctors' appointments
- Housekeeping
- Shopping (food, house supplies, medications, gifts)
- Sharing your feelings
- Unexpected problems (broken car, leaking freezer, etc.)

Depending upon your past experience with cancer, other people may be able to help you by:

- Getting information about your cancer and treatment
- Being a reader (someone who can read the information provided to you and research any additional information provided in pamphlets, books, and on the Internet)

- Being a listener (someone who can accompany you to your appointments and listen to all the questions and answers)
- Finding out about home health care, if needed

How do I ask for help?

Many people feel uncomfortable asking for help. Having cancer is not a usual circumstance. This is a most appropriate time to ask for help. When people call to offer to do something specific, such as picking up a prescription, say "yes." If they call and offer general help by asking, "Can I do anything?" tell them the specific things on your list. If they cannot help with any of these things at this time, tell them that their concern is appreciated and that you will contact them should any new needs arise. (Note: You do not owe it to anyone to share the details of your medical situation just because he or she helped out.)

How long will I need help?

Depending on your medical and personal situations, you may need help for many months. Let people know how long you think you might need help. Let them know when you still need help, especially if longer than originally planned. Otherwise, people might disappear from the helping scene simply because they are unaware that your need still exists.

Many people want to help and are able to help. Give them the opportunity to help by making your needs known.

Where do I ask for help?

Family and close friends are usually aware of your illness and will let you know if they can help. If you are part of a religious congregation, consider letting them know your situation. You may find yourself with offers from casual acquaintances and even strangers. Social or athletic organizations may also have members who are able to help. Many local and national volunteer support groups provide information and hands-on help. Doctors, nurses, and hospital social workers are familiar with organizations that provide services.

What if I'm receiving lots of phone calls?

Phone calls are wonderful when they help you to accept and adjust to the ups and downs of your illness, and when you feel comforted and inspired. Phone calls can become draining, though, even when your news is good. You may find yourself repeating the same stories over and over as well-wishers call to check on you. Phone calls can deplete your physical or emotional reserves, or keep you from getting jobs done or getting the rest you need. Your top priority is getting well, not keeping everyone else informed or happy.

How do I cut down the number of phone calls without hurting anybody's feelings?

Appoint one spokesperson (or one for each circle of friends and family) to keep the rest informed about whatever specifics you want shared. Ask everyone to call your spokesperson(s) instead of you when they want to send news or wishes or want updates.

Let people know if letters and e-mail messages are better than phone calls. Advantages include:

- You can read their messages when it's a good time for you, emotionally or physically.
- You can read messages again and again, including at those times when you need the contact but wouldn't call, such as 3 A.M.
- You regain a sense of control by choosing when you read your messages.
- The messages help you combat loneliness and feel connected to your friends and family.
- You can communicate with people who are far away, or who have colds or other infectious illnesses that prevent visits.

Managing the practical problems that arise during your evaluation and treatment will help you get good care. Knowing how to use the medical system will help, too, and is the topic of the next chapter.

4

Using the Medical System

Just as the medicine of cancer diagnosis and treatment is changing every year, so is the medical system in which doctors make the diagnoses and administer the treatments. Managed care is affecting how medicine is practiced in all hospitals and physicians' offices. Understanding the medical system in general, and your health plan in particular, will help you get the medical care you want and need.

YOUR PHYSICIANS

If I do not have an oncologist (cancer specialist), do I need one?

Generally speaking, yes. An **oncologist** who oversees your evaluation and treatment can help assure that you are getting state-of-the-art cancer care. Oncologists are experienced in preventing and managing the problems that can be seen in cancer patients. If you have a type of cancer that can be treated by an internist or family practitioner, get a recommendation about treatment from an oncologist before you begin your cancer therapy.

Most people with cancer are treated by one or more oncologists, such as:

- A medical oncologist—an internist specializing in cancer
- A radiation oncologist—a doctor trained to use radiation to diagnose and treat cancer
- A gynecologic oncologist—a gynecologist specializing in cancer
- A surgical oncologist—a surgeon specializing in cancer

What factors should I consider when choosing an oncologist?

You can learn about a doctor's credentials by checking the *American Medical Directory* or the *Directory of American Specialists* at your local library. If a doctor is Board Certified, he or she passed tests after completing training requirements. Good credentials and reputation are essential, but you'll also consider other factors when choosing a doctor, including:

- The doctor's experience in diagnosing and treating your type of cancer
- If the doctor is covered by your insurance plan (you can find this out by asking the doctor's office or calling the insurance company)
- How well you communicate and how comfortable you feel with the doctor
- The location of the doctor's office
- The hospital(s) with which the doctor is affiliated (the hospital to which the doctor admits his or her patients—see page 142)

How do I decide if a doctor is a good choice for me?

An effective doctor-patient relationship is vital. Although many different people can offer you comfort and support, only your physician can provide expert medical advice about effective therapies for treating your cancer. Only your physician can get you access to these therapies. You are probably making a good choice if all the following apply:

- The doctor is well-qualified in the treatment of your type of cancer.

- You trust your doctor's advice.
- You trust your doctor's concern for you as a person.
- You feel you can be honest, and you would be willing to inform your doctor about your pain, anxiety, depression, and so on.

You may be most comfortable in a collegial sort of relationship with your physicians. Or, you may be best served when your physicians assume a more paternalistic role. Some superb clinicians like to make jokes or tell stories while examining patients; others do their job best when they are strictly business. There is no one right or best way for doctors and patients to relate to each other. The relationship doesn't have to be perfect, either, for it to work well.

The world's most famous and respected physician for your type of cancer may not be the best physician *for you* if your personality styles clash, you simply can't communicate well, or the doctor can't see you for a few weeks. Make your needs clear to your doctor before you decide that he or she is not right for you. Working with a doctor is a two-way association, and sometimes it takes a few visits before a good rapport develops. Weeks or months that you spend looking for the ideal doctor-patient relationship is time away from healing relationships with doctors who are available to you.

An effective doctor-patient relationship is one in which you and your doctor work together toward a common goal: getting you well as surely, safely, easily, and quickly as possible.

Do I have to ask my doctor lots of questions?

Informed patients can participate more effectively in their care. If you don't understand something, ask. If you think something might be amiss such as a test that was ordered or a medication that was prescribed, ask! You have a right to understand your care and protect yourself if you think something isn't right.

Some books and articles on survivorship make it seem as if you have to become a medical expert and question everything your doctors say and do in order to maximize the quality of your care. Actually, this approach may hamper the healing process by making it hard for you to relax and trust the care you receive. Incessant questioning may make it harder for your doctors to do their job well, too. To be informed means to know *enough, not everything.*

Try to find a realistic balance between how many medical details you need to understand and what you leave to your doctors. Then, find doctors who can match your style. For example, if you like to read the medical literature and ask a lot of questions, you'll be happiest with a doctor who respects this need and helps you get the information you desire. Alternatively, if you want to be relieved of any responsibility for sorting through the medical options, you need a doctor who is comfortable just giving you recommendations without much explanation.

Who makes the final decision about my treatment — my physicians or me?

You. No matter how much or little you choose to learn about your illness, and no matter how strong your doctors' opinions, your doctors only make recommendations. You decide whether to follow them or not. Physicians' recommendations are based on their fund of knowledge and experience, professional interpretation of your medical situation, and concern for you as a person. They provide a valuable objectivity when guiding you.

Why does it matter with whom my doctor shares responsibility for patients?

Almost all doctors share responsibility for patients with other doctors. "Call" is slang for "duty." During weekends, holidays, and possibly weekday evenings, many doctors rotate who is "on call" and therefore who is responsible for patient care. On the days when your doctor is not on call, you can expect to be cared for by the doctor who is on duty should an emergency come up or if you are in the hospital.

Some doctors participate in a team practice. This means that instead of having one primary doctor, all the doctors share equally in your care. Since having cancer involves a long-term relationship with your doctors, you might consider getting to know some or all the other doctors who will take care of you.

Does it matter to what hospital my doctor admits his or her patients?

Yes. Hospital affiliation is one factor that may influence your choice of oncologist. Although, in general, oncologists admit their patients only to hospitals that are well equipped to care for cancer patients, some differences exist among hospitals that may be important to you such as:

- Availability of special services such as stem-cell transplantation, gamma-knife radiation, or stereotactic radiation implants
- Involvement with cancer research (researchers are involved with the latest advances)
- Size (there are advantages and disadvantages to both small community hospitals and large comprehensive cancer centers)
- Coverage by your insurance policy
- Location (families have an easier time visiting and helping when you are close by)

If you want or need your oncologist to be involved any time you are hospitalized, you will have to be in a hospital where he or she has admitting privileges. This could be a problem if this hospital is not covered by your insurance or is far from your home. Keep in mind that even if you are scheduled for all outpatient cancer treatments, there is always the possibility that you will need to be hospitalized to treat a cancer-related problem or something totally unrelated to your cancer treatments such as appendicitis. In an emergency, you can be evaluated and treated at another hospital by other doctors until you are discharged home or are well enough to be transferred to your oncologist's hospital.

Although it is not necessary for good care, you may prefer to have all your doctors affiliated with one hospital. Communication among doctors may be easier when they all work together at one institution, and you may find it more convenient or comforting to go for checkups and treatments in the same general location. If you have this desire, find out about your doctors' hospital affiliations.

What is a Comprehensive Cancer Center?

Comprehensive Cancer Centers are accredited and supported by the National Cancer Institute for integrating strong basic, clinical, prevention, control, and population sciences. Forty centers in the United States meet the strict criteria for being designated a Comprehensive Cancer Center. They all provide a variety of services, including standard cancer treatments (chemotherapy, radiation therapy, immunotherapy), counseling, rehabilitation, nutritional counseling, home-care supervision, outreach, and education. Most have research and teaching facilities and staff.

In addition to the accredited Comprehensive Cancer Centers, twelve Clinical Cancer Centers are funded in part by the National Cancer Institute. These centers conduct cancer research and provide training programs in addition to state-of-the-art cancer care. You can call the toll-free cancer-information service (800-4-CANCER) or go to www3.cancer.gov/cancercenters/centerslist.html for a list of NCI-designated Comprehensive Cancer Centers and Clinical Cancer Centers. Note that some for-profit institutions call themselves cancer centers or comprehensive cancer centers.

Do I need to be evaluated at a major cancer center?

Well-meaning people may urge you to go to a major cancer center such as the M. D. Anderson Cancer Center in Houston or the Memorial Sloan-Kettering Cancer Center in New York. The advantages are:

- Doctors at these centers have considerable experience with all types of cancer, including rare cancers.
- These centers offer investigational programs (clinical trials).
- These centers offer state-of-the-art evaluation and treatment.

The disadvantages are:

- It can be expensive, not only in terms of dollars but also in terms of time, travel, and emotional energy.
- It may require separation from your family and support network.

- A doctor referral may be needed to set up an appointment and/or for your insurance to cover the evaluation.
- The evaluation may feel less personal and you may feel like "a number."

Sometimes, your local doctors can discuss your case over the phone with specialists at the major cancer centers. As a result, in some cases it is not necessary for you to travel to the cancer center. Your doctor can advise you whether or not a trip is worthwhile.

INSURANCE

What should I do if my oncologist is not on my health plan?

When possible, try to establish yourself with a reputable doctor who is covered by your insurance plan, possibly one recommended by your current doctor. But even this precaution has limits; many doctors and employers switch plans from year to year.

If you want to see a physician who is outside your plan, find out from your insurance company or your doctor whether you can be reimbursed for at least a portion of the fees, or whether the doctor provides any special expertise or service that would qualify for coverage under your plan. Ask whether your doctor can or will become part of your plan; but remember that voiced intentions are not commitments.

If you have a "point-of-service" option, you can choose to go to health-care providers outside your plan, usually for an additional fee. If your plan will not reimburse at all for a particular oncologist's services, and if you can afford it, you may want to invest in a one-time consultation for a second opinion regarding your diagnosis and treatment. Often, choosing a course of treatment is the critical task that requires the most experienced judgment; administering the treatments may be straightforward and routine at any oncology office.

If you want to see an out-of-plan oncologist throughout your treatment, you will have to balance the value of seeing this particular doctor against the hardship of paying bills out-of-pocket.

Your doctor's office can predict visit fees and estimate total doctor charges. The *actual* cost to you will depend on your medical course and the outcome of your treatments. Bills can mount up quickly if you develop problems or complications that require hospitalization or extra visits—a not uncommon situation even with ultimately successful treatment. It is best to avoid the stress of having to choose between incurring burdensome debts and switching oncologists in the middle of treatment. Explain your financial situation to your doctor and the staff in charge of billing. Open communication, including a willingness to show them your income tax returns, increases the chance that they can arrange delayed or reduced payments.

Keep in mind that qualified oncologists are well equipped to diagnose and treat most types of cancer. Not everyone needs to be treated by the most famous oncologists or at the most prestigious institutions. The financial advantages to you of staying within your plan must be balanced against the psychological and medical advantages of going outside your plan.

What if my oncologist advises a stem-cell transplant and my insurance company denies covering it?

Proceed with your appointment for consultation with the medical team at the transplant center. Most centers are experienced with filing appeals and persuading insurers to cover the cost. Attorneys, especially those experienced in getting insurers to pay for transplants, can file an appeal with supporting evidence and ask the insurer to reconsider the claim. *The Blood & Marrow Transplant Newsletter* (2900 Skokie Valley Road, Suite B, Highland Park, IL 60035; 847-433-3133, 888-597-7674; www.bmtnews.org) provides referral to attorneys with success in appealing denials of stem-cell transplants. If your attorney does not have special expertise in this area, you might want to reserve the right to supplement your appeal at a later date. Involving your local politicians might bring influential attention to your personal situation, and allow you to voice your concerns to policy makers.

When transplant offers you the best chance at long-term survival, get the treatment you need now. Later, you can worry about paying for your treatments or pushing to change your insurance company's guidelines.

What if I don't understand my entitlements under my current policy?

If you are unclear about any aspects of your policy, you can bring your questions and concerns to:

- Your insurer
- Your state's Department of Insurance, which may be listed in your telephone directory under "Insurance Department," "Division of Insurance," "Office of Insurance," "Commerce and Economic Development Department," "Division of Consumer Affairs," or "Bureau of Consumer Assistance"
- Your oncologist's billing office or office manager
- Your hospital's billing office or office of patient affairs
- The American Cancer Society (ask for their booklet "Cancer Treatments Your Insurance Should Cover")
- The National Coalition for Cancer Survivorship (ask for their booklet "What Cancer Survivors Need to Know About Health Insurance")

What about the stories of people in managed care receiving inferior cancer care?

After a cancer diagnosis, your priority must be getting the care you need, whether it is in your managed-care plan or not. Ideally, all your needs and preferences can be met within the restrictions imposed by your plan. If you are uncomfortable with your current doctor, try switching to another doctor within your plan. If your plan does not cover payment for a service or treatment that you consider your first choice (medically, emotionally, or logistically), you may have to compromise. You may have to bear the financial burden of out-of-pocket payments or accept one of your lower choices of physicians, hospitals, or reasonable treatment options. This may happen if your plan restricts access to:

- The individual physicians you prefer to see
- Specific treatments, such as investigational drugs, devices, or treatments or "off-label" use of chemotherapies (used when your type of cancer is not listed on the package insert)
- Treatment at certain hospitals

If you believe that you are being denied an optimal evaluation or treatment, complain to your insurance providers. Your grievances may not be heard for a month or two. While waiting for a response from your health plan, pursue your search for the best treatment for you. If you need a test or treatment that your plan won't cover, go outside the plan. Don't let a bureaucracy prohibit you from getting the care you deserve.

Don't fail to act. Be proactive in using your health plan.

How do I start dealing with my insurance claims?

It is very important that you keep your current policies in force by paying all required premiums on time and in full. Obtaining new insurance after you have been diagnosed with cancer can be difficult and expensive.

- Make sure your premiums are up-to-date! Don't lose your insurance coverage because your bill sits unpaid on your desk while you get evaluated.
- Obtain a copy of the most current plan booklet from your insurance carrier.
- Obtain some blank insurance claim forms.
- Make a copy of everything that you submit for payment.
- Make a copy of all communications to insurance companies.
- Keep the Explanation of Benefits form (EOB) together with your copy of the claim form and invoice.
- Review your bills for accuracy; review what has been paid by your insurance company. (Errors do occur.)
- Submit claims for everything for which you are billed, including wigs and medications.
- File claims on time. You may forfeit your right to reimburse-

ment if you don't file within twelve months or in the same calendar year of the service.

- If a claim is denied and you feel that this is in error, have the doctor's office and the insurance company advise you about how to pursue reimbursement.
- Check to see if you have a Waiver of Premium feature. If so, you don't have to pay premiums during the time of illness or disability.
- Your doctors' offices and the insurance company can help advise you about which bills probably will be covered by your insurance.

Is there anything that I can do if my claim is denied?

Yes. If your insurance company denies payment on a claim and you are sure the denial is not justified, do not give up! Resubmit the claim. If denied again, be persistent. Ask for a review. If still denied, request a review by the peer review physicians. Claims that are rejected the first time often are paid the second time around. Some must be resubmitted four or five times before being approved. Have your doctor's office help you if you feel a legitimate claim was denied. If you still have trouble, you can go through the appeals process with the assistance of your state's insurance commissioner. In a large, bureaucratic organization such as an insurance company, the squeaky wheel gets the grease.

What is precertification?

Precertification is approval by a representative of the insurance company *before* you receive a specific medical service or, in the case of an emergency, within a given number of hours or days. Your insurance company may require precertification for full reimbursement. For example, you may have to call an 800 telephone number provided by your insurer before proceeding with a scan, biopsy, second opinion, or elective hospitalization. If you don't get precertification, the insurance company can deny part or all of the reimbursement, even if they agree with the need for the service.

Make sure you know which services require precertification. Give the precertification instructions to family members or friends so that they can get proper approval if, for some reason, you can't do it.

Where can I go for more information or help with my insurance?

"What Cancer Survivors Need to Know About Health Insurance" is an excellent booklet published by the National Coalition for Cancer Survivorship. After explaining the various types of insurance and reviewing the basics about Medicare, it offers advice about:

- Obtaining or continuing health insurance
- Maximizing coverage for investigational therapies
- Handling claims that are denied
- Other resources

Is there anyone who can help me file claims with my insurance company?

Yes. Most major cities have professional claim-filing services or consultants—called (medical) claims adjusters, consulters, or assistants—that you can hire to file your bills. Given the larger claims common for cancer care, it is money well spent. Fees range from $25 to $75 per hour or operate on a commission of 10 percent of recovered funds, and are usually negotiable. Most contested claims can be resolved with less than ten hours of professional time. Consultants can offer tips for managing claims that minimize the amount of professional time you would need to get the job done.

Look in the Yellow Pages under "Insurance Claim (or 'Medical Claim') Processing Services." Note that some of these services are for physicians' offices only. Major insurance companies sometimes have a delegated carrier representative (sometimes called a "care coordinator") who will file for patients and/or work with them on their medical claims. Referrals to a service might be obtained from your physician, family lawyer, accountant, membership group (community-based or religion-affiliated organization), corporate-benefits department at your place of work, or the social-service department at your local hospital.

Why would I want to employ a consultant to file my medical bills?

Hiring a consultant can save you money when medical bills seem unfair but are too complex for you to understand or talk about, or when you've contested claims without success. Even if you are not involved in a last-ditch effort to pay your bills, consultants may be worthwhile for you because they

- can relieve you of some of the emotional stress associated with slogging through mounds of bills;
- can free up some time (money well spent when your time feels stretched to the limit);
- may pick up improper charges that you missed, especially on complex or costly charges.

Why would I want a financial counselor?

Even if you have good medical insurance, the nonmedical costs may strain your resources. Expenses that often are not reimbursed include transportation to and from treatments, child care, housekeepers, nurse's aides, and many treatment-related products, such as nutritional supplements or prostheses (artificial body parts or aids). In addition, your household may be experiencing a significant loss of income because you or the other wage earners in your home have to take time off without pay to tend to your needs.

Financial counselors help you plan your budget. Look in the telephone book under "Consumer Credit Counseling Services." Nonprofit services may provide free or low-cost assistance; for-profit services will charge a fee. For more information, or assistance locating a nonprofit service, contact the National Foundation for Credit Counseling on line at: www.nfcc.org. Member offices can be reached in communities nationwide by calling toll-free 800-388-2227.

What if costs are a strain on my family's finances?

Cancer can be a very expensive illness, even when your treatments are covered by insurance. You may have too many assets to qualify for public financial support, yet be struggling with rising bills as you experience a loss in income related to your illness. Accepting financial support or free services may be difficult for you, especially if you've always taken care of your own needs. By accepting assistance, you can better focus your energy on getting well. Learn about people and organizations that provide services and funds to families in need whether they qualify for public aid or not. Some organizations to contact include:

- The American Cancer Society—most local chapters have programs providing wigs, hospital beds, wheelchairs, and other noncovered essentials, as well as transportation to and from treatment centers and doctors' offices (when volunteers are available)
- Local chapters of other cancer organizations such as Y-Me, Us-Too, Leukemia and Lymphoma Society of America, Let's Face It, and so on
- Religious organizations and communities
- Community service organizations
- Social-services department of your local hospital
- Local public-assistance office
- Cancer support groups such as Wellness Communities and Gilda's Clubs
- Social, work, and school organizations
- Pharmaceutical companies that offer free or reduced-cost drugs to those in financial need

What if I don't qualify for aid but I can't afford the cancer care I feel I need to get well?

Until health-care reform makes this question irrelevant, you can minimize how much money you borrow or take out of your savings for cancer treatment by

- discussing with your doctors all the treatment options for your illness, and their estimated costs;
- being open with your health-care team about your financial concerns so that you can be informed about any flexibility in payment schedules;
- finding out about all services that are available to people in your situation;
- finding out if you are eligible for free or reduced-rate medications from pharmaceutical companies;
- contacting a financial counselor;
- taking the proper deductions for medical expenses from your federal income taxes (call the Internal Revenue Service for information).

What if I don't have any medical insurance?

Your options for obtaining medical insurance may be limited and expensive, but there are still steps you can take to ease the financial burden of cancer care. You can look into a high-risk pool, or an individual policy with certain limitations, but these tend to be prohibitively expensive. In some states, large corporations are required to insure you.

You can learn about your rights and options (they differ from state to state) from current publications. Since laws and policies are changing, information and advice may become outdated quickly. Confirm and supplement what you learn from books with information and advice from:

- National Coalition for Cancer Survivorship (www .canceradvocacy.org) or other advocacy organizations
- Your state's insurance and welfare departments
- Patient-services organizations
- A financial planner experienced in health care
- An attorney experienced in health care

Even without medical insurance, there are steps you can take to get medical care. You may qualify for Medicaid if you are low income. You may qualify for Medicare or Social Security benefits if you are:

- Totally disabled and have been collecting Social Security benefits for at least twenty-four months
- Legally blind
- On renal dialysis
- Sixty-five years or older and entitled to Social Security, widow's, or railroad retirement benefits

There may be local organizations that provide free or reduced-rate health care to those in financial hardship. Many people have sponsored successful drives to raise money for patients who needed expensive treatments and who didn't have adequate insurance.

Can I be fired from my job if I need to take time off for treatment?

No, not if your employer is covered by a state or federal law that prohibits discrimination against people with disabilities. Under the Family and Medical Leave Act of 1993, employers with at least fifty employees are required to allow up to twelve weeks of unpaid medical leave for treatment or to care for a legal dependent. During this period, your health-insurance benefits must continue without interruption. The Americans with Disabilities Act prohibits employers with at least fifteen employees from firing you if you need a limited amount of time off as a "reasonable accommodation." Some state laws offer even more protection from discrimination.

Am I going to be able to get insurance if I switch jobs or start my own business?

People can feel locked into their current jobs after a diagnosis of cancer because of problems getting insurance if they switch jobs. As of July 1, 1997, the Health Insurance Reform Act protects you by

- prohibiting insurers from denying coverage or charging higher premiums to individuals *in group plans* because of their medical history or status;
- prohibiting insurers from imposing preexisting-condition exclusions for more than twelve months for any condition

diagnosed or treated in the preceding six months (you may have to cover expenses for your cancer-related care for twelve months, at most);

- prohibiting insurers from imposing any preexisting-condition exclusion on an individual who has already had the allowed twelve-month exclusion and who has maintained continuous coverage (namely, no more than a sixty-three-day gap in coverage);
- assuring availability of individual policies for those who are fired or leave jobs voluntarily and for their dependents as long as they have maintained continuous private coverage for the preceding eighteen months and are ineligible for further coverage under COBRA (Comprehensive Omnibus Budget Reconciliation Act);
- prohibiting insurers from refusing to sell plans to small employers with two to fifty employees.

Unfortunately, you still may have problems because

- insurers may comply with the act by offering policies that are prohibitively expensive;
- the protection against preexisting-condition exclusions does not apply to those covered by individual (versus group) policies;
- the protections do not apply to mental-health coverage;
- the protections do not help the uninsured.

Explore all your options. Discuss insurance problems with your physicians and with the support staff at the hospital.

Asking for assistance provides an opportunity for others to feel fulfilled. Accepting help promotes your recovery.

Why is talking about insurance so emotional?

Talking about the financial burden of your cancer care can be highly emotional for you and those who care about you. Many people find it easier to talk about anything, even their death, than to discuss their money issues. If you feel very emotional, it may be because you

- regret some decisions you made about what insurance you purchased;
- feel guilty about tapping into family savings to pay for your care;
- feel angry, sad, or confused about the financial burden being added to all the other losses accompanying your illness;
- feel the uncertainty and seriousness surrounding your illness as you talk in the more concrete terms of dollars and cents.

Talking openly about your insurance and financial concerns will help you understand what is happening and make wise decisions.

WILLS/LIVING WILLS

Do I need to do anything about my will?

Everyone needs a will, whether they have cancer or not. Make sure that your will is up-to-date. Also make sure that family, friends, or your physicians know where your will is kept. If you do not have a will, you should obtain a lawyer and create one now, particularly if

- you are very ill;
- you are going to undergo high-risk surgery or a high-risk procedure;
- you are not very ill and you feel that you can handle it emotionally.

Do I really need to think about a will right now?

Tending to your will does not mean in any way that you are going to die soon or that you think that you might die soon. Simply put, everyone should have an updated will at all times so that if anything should happen, such as a fatal car accident or heart attack, those left behind would handle our affairs the way we would like. A well-written will minimizes problems for those tending to our affairs and decreases the amount of funds lost to taxes.

A will is a sensitive issue to discuss, especially if you have just been diagnosed with cancer. If you are struggling with your new diagnosis, it may be difficult and emotionally damaging to bring up the emotionally charged issue of a will. If you are unsure whether you or your family can handle a discussion of your will, have your doctor or a hospital social worker give you and your family some guidance on how to deal with this matter.

What if I'm worried that preparing my will means I've given up hope?

Making a will, even preparing for your own funeral, does not mean that you have given up hope or are pessimistic about your future. Paradoxically, taking care of your will may free you to have strong hope for a complete recovery by taking care of the "What ifs?" that may otherwise nag at you at one level or another. Preparing a will is like buying fire insurance: It causes anxiety while you do it but thereafter offers peace of mind. Once you've completed the paperwork, you are less worried about disasters because you've taken the steps you can take to protect yourself.

Preparing a will may free you to have strong hope for your recovery by decreasing some worries.

What is a medical proxy?

A medical "**proxy**" or "agent" is an adult whom you assign to assume legal authority to make life-and-death decisions for you in the event that you are unable to make them for yourself. Most people choose a close family member or friend who knows your wishes and is willing to carry them out. The legal document that allows you to transfer your right to make health decisions is called a "**durable power of attorney**." Assigning a proxy and preparing a durable power of attorney are the best ways to ensure that your wishes will be carried out.

What is a living will?

A living will is a written statement that outlines what you would or would not like done to prolong your life artificially should recovery become almost impossible. This document can be written when a person is totally healthy or after an illness has occurred. You must be considered legally able (i.e., competent) to sign a living will. A living will is not as effective or binding as a durable power of attorney (see above question).

The Self-Determination Act of 1991 deemed that patients be informed about their rights under state law to accept or refuse treatment; it also helps patients execute a living will and appoint a medical proxy if they so wish. You can obtain more information and/or a blank form from your doctor, your lawyer, or from:

Partnership for Caring—America's Voices for the Dying
1620 Eye Street NW, Suite 202
Washington, DC 20006
800-989-9455
www.partnershipforcaring.org

OBTAINING MORE MEDICAL INFORMATION

What additional information do I need?

Sound information helps you get the best medical care possible. It also helps you minimize the physical and emotional pain, debility, and loss due to your cancer and its treatment. Everyone has an individual style and a unique need for information. As you go through your treatments, you may find yourself dealing with new medical, emotional, practical, social, spiritual, or financial problems. Depending upon your situation, you may need or desire additional information about

- your type of cancer and treatments;
- your treatment options, including clinical trials, if your current treatment isn't working well;
- how to make wise choices, medical and otherwise;
- how to get assistance, medical and otherwise;
- the nonmedical issues of survivorship.

You help yourself when you learn enough to help your healthcare team take good care of you during your treatments. Depending upon your medical course, you may do fine with what you learned during the first few weeks. Or, you may do best by continuing your cancer education throughout your treatments. As you near the end of your treatments, learning about the medical, practical, and emotional issues that arise after completion of treatments may help make your recovery and long-term survivorship as smooth and healing as possible.

What if medical information just makes me feel anxious or confused?

You don't need to become a quasi-expert on cancer to be an effective patient. Attempts to grasp the complex science of oncology may cause you to feel overwhelmed and even more out of control. You need to know *enough,* not everything. Usually, the information about your disease and treatment offered by your doctors and nurses, and supplemented by pamphlets for patients, provides enough medical background. You are doing well if you can learn what you must know to

- help your doctors take care of you (see chapter 3),
- do what helps you get better between office visits, and
- avoid things that hurt you.

Let your family and health-care team know how much medical information you can handle right now. How much you can learn and how much you want to learn may vary over time. You may want to learn more later

Am I hurting my chances if I don't learn a lot about cancer?

The main advantages of learning about your cancer are that you can

- participate in the decision making;
- possibly find a reasonable treatment option not presented by your doctors;
- be tuned in to problems when they are early, and take steps to minimize them;
- understand more of what is happening.

Knowledge can help you advocate for yourself in a meaningful way and reinforce your confidence that you are getting the best care possible. If you feel that you want this sense of personal advocacy but don't have the time or strength to amass the information yourself, you can have trusted family members or friends do the medical research for you and advise you on all the medical decisions that arise throughout your treatment and recovery.

Where can I obtain additional information?
- Libraries (public and medical)
- Local, state, and national organizations
- Cancer centers
- Your doctors' offices
- Reputable Internet sites
- Bookstores
- Other survivors

How do I find out about local and national organizations?
- Look in the Yellow Pages under your type of cancer.
- Call the American Cancer Society for a listing.
- Call or write to the National Coalition for Cancer Survivorship.
- Surf the Internet.

What about the Internet?
The Internet is becoming an increasingly useful tool for obtaining and sharing information about all aspects of survivorship, including:

- Medical information
- Clinical trials
- Support organizations
- Pain management
- Financial information
- Announcements of upcoming meetings and conferences
- Cancer publications
- Mailing lists for specific types of cancer, or specific needs
- On-line support groups

A personal computer with access to the Internet allows you to obtain information in the privacy of your home, participate in an on-line support group, listen to a Web cast, put your name on mailing lists for survivors, and contact physicians and other health-care professionals who respond to questions on line.

Libraries often have free access to the Internet, inexpensive printing charges, and support staff to help you obtain needed information. Find a friend or relative who knows the Internet and is willing to surf cyberspace for you.

Is all the information on the Internet reliable?

No. Anyone can publish to the World Wide Web. Much of the information and advice is inaccurate and some of it is dangerous even when it is presented in scientific-sounding terms. It is important to know which Web sites offer true, accurate, reliable, and up-to-date information. Interlinked sites are not always of equal quality. Whenever information differs at all from what you've been told, discuss it with your doctors.

Don't trust everything you read on the Internet.

How do I get started on the Internet?

Go to the Web site of the National Coalition for Cancer Survivorship at www.canceradvocacy.org. You've now accessed "Cansearch: A Guide to Cancer Resources on the Internet," courtesy of the National Coalition for Cancer Survivorship, which can guide you through the other resources for cancer survivors and provide nearly unlimited links.

What if I'm having a hard time?

Knowing about your disease and treatment and how to be an effective patient helps you get good medical care. But this knowledge alone doesn't eliminate the stress and strain. The next chapter will discuss the emotional side of the first few months. You'll read about taming your fears, understanding the wide variety of feelings you and your family may experience, and knowing how to relate to others or how to help your children adjust to the changes. Learning about the emotional aspects of a cancer diagnosis will help you get good care and live as fully as possible during treatment.

5

—

The Emotional Adjustment

A diagnosis of cancer can be as much an emotional as a physical challenge. You and your loved ones may find yourselves experiencing a wide variety of feelings. If extreme, feelings can contribute to your sense of unreality or confusion. They can cause tremendous inner stress and can strain your relationships with others. This chapter will introduce you to the emotional aspects of dealing with cancer. Learning what to expect will help you know that you aren't going crazy, and know when and where to get assistance, if needed. This chapter will encourage you to use your emotions in healing ways.

FEELINGS

How am I supposed to feel?

There is no right way to feel after you have been told you have cancer. Whatever you feel is the right way for you. Common, normal feelings and reactions include:

- Fear
- Crying
- Sense of unreality

- Sense of loss of control
- Loneliness
- Anger
- Panic
- Confusion
- Irrational thoughts
- Poor concentration and difficulty making decisions
- Irritability
- Change in appetite
- Diminished or absent sexual drive
- Change in sleeping pattern; nightmares

You may have none, some, or all these feelings and reactions. The feelings may be vague and mild, or clear and extreme. They can come and go. These reactions are your body's way of adjusting to the news. Some of your feelings can be due to, or exacerbated by, your medications.

What does it mean if I'm experiencing a lot of emotions?

Your emotions are

- the signal of a change or problem, or
- the reaction to a change or problem.

Feeling anxious may be due to fear of pain, future debility, or dying. Feeling sad may be part of your grief reaction to losing your health, a body part, or plans for the immediate future. Anger may arise if you believe your diagnosis was delayed because earlier complaints were ignored, or if you are now feeling abandoned by friends or family. You will not feel like this forever; these intense emotions will lessen with time. Whatever you are feeling inside, be sure that you continue to get medical attention during this adjustment phase.

What should I do if I have strong emotions?

Let your feelings and reactions happen. Talk about them with friends, family, your nurse, or a cancer support group. Try to find someone who has been through a similar experience and who can help you sort through the problems that are generating or fueling your emotions. Write about your reactions and feelings in a diary or a letter. Professional counseling may be enormously beneficial, enabling you to get through your evaluation and treatment more quickly and with less emotional distress than if you tried to work through your feelings on your own. Counseling is available from nurse therapists, clinical social workers, psychologists, psychiatrists, and clergypersons.

Being told you have cancer is a major event in your life. What thoughts and feelings you have are not as important as what you do with them.

Is it unhealthy for me to feel emotional?

No. Having many or powerful emotions is not a problem *unless*

- your emotions keep you from getting good medical care;
- you try to hide your unpleasant emotions all the time;
- you try to fight or deny unpleasant feelings;
- your emotions keep you from relating to your physicians, nurses, family, or friends;
- your emotions prevent you from eating or sleeping.

Unpleasant emotions are not the problem; they are the signal of a problem or your body's response to a problem.

What if I am having trouble believing that this is really happening?

It is common for people with a new diagnosis of cancer to say, "I cannot believe that this is happening" or " I feel like this is all a bad dream and I'm going to wake up." This is the numbing effect of shock, and it's normal. Numbness or a sense of unreality protects you from the full emotional impact of your diagnosis while still allowing you to begin the process of getting medical care. This reaction can last days or even months. If it lasts longer than that, you may need some help to move on with your adjustment.

Even if you are experiencing disbelief, you still must proceed with getting attention for your cancer. If your reactions seem overwhelming, if you can't make decisions, or if you can't bring yourself to get medical attention, have your doctor direct you to people or support groups who can help you through this early adjustment phase. Having trouble believing this is really happening is normal. Denying that this is happening (or denying that you need to do anything about it) is not normal, and heals nobody.

What if my treatment plan seems overwhelming?

Just as a successful jogger runs a marathon one mile at a time, think about getting through the first week of radiation or the first cycle of chemotherapy (or the first dose, if that works better for you.) When a series of different treatments is planned, try to concentrate on the treatment segment you are facing now. For example, try to push the planned subsequent surgery or radiation therapy out of your mind until you are almost done with your current chemotherapy. It may help to find out if there is anything you can do to prepare for your next treatment. This encourages you to think about future treatments only in terms of what you can do about them now.

Another technique that may help is to plan a special event to mark the end of each phase of treatment. In this way you can focus on the anticipated pleasurable commemoration. Be sure to think of something easy and dependable, such as watching a favorite movie on TV with a special friend or tearing up the calendar page on which you've been crossing off the days of treatment.

What if I feel uncomfortable saying the word "cancer"?

"Cancer" is a very emotional word for some people. It is common to have difficulty saying the word "cancer" at first because of all the frightening things that you associate with this disease. The right way to handle this is whatever feels comfortable for you. Find the word or phrase that you find easiest to say now (e.g., "tumor," "malignancy," "problem"). Do what is comfortable for you, not for other people. If you are not yet ready to use the word "cancer," don't!

Many people find that the more they use the word "cancer," the less and less emotional or scary it becomes. "Cancer" becomes just one more regular word in your vocabulary. Other people may be offended or uncomfortable if you say "cancer" frequently. That's their problem, not yours.

What if I feel sad?

The human reaction to loss is grief—a heavy feeling in the chest, mental distress, and a sense of emptiness or sadness. If you feel sad, acknowledge the many little and big losses that may be causing you to feel this way: your health, a body part or function, your normal energy, thwarted plans or dreams, your job or insurance, time flexibility (cancer treatment can be very time-consuming), friends, privacy (having cancer can make you a public figure in your social circles), and so on.

Express your sadness; share it with people who understand and care. Sometimes it is hard for your loved ones to absorb your grief or respond in a helpful way because, for example, they may feel the need to keep your spirits up at all times. In these cases, sharing with objective third parties such as counselors or clergy is invaluable. Even when family and friends are good listeners and comforters, professionals are experienced in dealing with a new diagnosis and can provide pearls of wisdom that complement the comfort offered by people more closely involved in your life.

When you feel the urge to cry, find a safe place to cry until you no longer feel the urge. If you're too embarrassed to cry, or the tears just won't come, watch a tear-jerker movie or play some music that touches your heartstrings and helps you cry. It takes energy to keep sadness inside, energy that can be better used toward healing and living the life you have.

Grieving helps you to adjust and leave the sadness behind as you move forward.

What if I feel depressed?

Depression is very different from sadness, even though people who are depressed usually feel sad. It has become commonplace to interchange the words "sad" and "depressed," as in "I'm really depressed that my shirt has a stain on it." "Depression" is a technical term that, in medical usage, refers to specific illnesses that can be diagnosed and treated.

"**Reactive depression**" is a common response to a cancer diagnosis and represents one way that helps many survivors adjust to the initial shock and changes. Reactive depression is a short-term, self-limited part of the grief process. "**Major depression**" (significant or long-lasting depression) is different from reactive depression. Although it often accompanies serious, chronic illness, depression is *not* an expected and normal part of having cancer. Just like pain or an infection, depression is a condition that needs medical attention, especially since it often improves or resolves with proper treatment.

How do I know if I am depressed?

Depression must be diagnosed by a trained professional. The diagnosis can be more difficult to make in the setting of cancer because many of the symptoms that help define depression can be due to cancer or its treatment, such as loss of appetite or sleep disturbance. Your physician may evaluate you for possible depression if, for at least two weeks, you have these three symptoms:

- Extreme feelings of sadness
- Loss of interest in people or activities that are important to you
- Loss of the ability to feel any pleasure

plus three or more of the following symptoms:

- Significant sleep problems (falling asleep, staying asleep, and/or nightmares)
- Change in appetite
- Fatigue, loss of energy
- Moving or thinking slowly
- Feeling agitated
- Feelings of worthlessness or guilt
- Poor concentration; difficulty making decisions
- Thoughts of suicide

Depression is a common medical problem. You may have a history of depression or a tendency toward depression that becomes activated in the setting of your illness. Some people who have never had emotional or psychiatric problems in their lives first experience depression after a cancer diagnosis.

Can my cancer cells be causing me to be depressed?

Certain types of cancer are associated with high rates of depression, such as (in decreasing order) pancreatic, mouth and pharynx, colon, breast, gynecologic, and lymphomas. Certain cancer treatments can, themselves, cause depression (for example, interferon) or lead to physical changes (for example, premature menopause) that increase the risk of depression. Whether your symptoms are due to your cancer, your treatment, something else, or the whole situation, you need to be evaluated to determine if you

- have depression and, if so, to define exactly what kind of depression;
- are receiving any treatments that are causing or exacerbating the depression and, if so, which can be stopped without compromising your recovery from cancer;
- would benefit from counseling and, if so, to define what type(s) would be best;
- would benefit from antidepressant medication and, if so, the best choice(s).

What if I am ashamed or embarrassed to tell my physician that I feel depressed?

There is tremendous social pressure to be a hero, a brave cancer warrior, and a stoic patient. If your doctors ask how you are, and you say, "Fine," when in fact you feel low, nothing will be done to help your situation. Your physicians can provide proper care for you only if you provide complete, honest information about all your symptoms, including those that suggest depression.

Diagnosing and treating depression requires honest communication between you and your physician.

Why is it important to determine if I have significant depression?

Diagnosing depression is important because depression

- is a painful condition that is treatable;
- may impair your overall health at a time when you need all your resources to get better;
- is associated with increased disability and length of hospitalization in medically ill patients;
- may make it difficult for you to comply with treatments, get good nutrition, or engage in adequate physical activity;
- diminishes your quality of life;
- is hard on those who care about you.

What if my family thinks that my mood reflects a negative attitude?

Attitude is a frame of mind. Serious depression is a medical condition in which your brain chemistry is out of balance. Attitude is a complex phenomenon, but it usually can be shaped voluntarily to a great degree. Depression is an illness, not a chosen outlook on life. Unless you want to be miserable, any significant depression you may be experiencing is not your fault. Depression deserves the same sympathy and medical attention as bleeding, vomiting, or any other medical problem.

As research unlocks some of the mysteries surrounding the chemistry of depression, the stigma surrounding this condition is fading. Unfortunately, friends, family members, or even some professionals may suggest that you're supposed to be depressed since you have cancer and, therefore, nothing needs to be evaluated or treated. Conversely, others may impatiently urge you to "Get a grip and cheer up!"

Find people who know how to diagnose and treat depression. If you are diagnosed with a reactive depression, all you may need is some time and emotional support. A brief course of medication may be indicated if, for example, the depression is keeping you from eating, sleeping, or getting care for your cancer. Or you may find out that what others are labeling "depression" is really a normal, healing grief process or the outward expression of a medical condition such as hypothyroidism (low thyroid levels). If you are found to be suffering from a major depression, appropriate treatment can be tried.

How is depression treated?

Once an accurate diagnosis has been made, your physicians will offer treatment options. Depression may resolve after your current medications are adjusted and you receive counseling regarding diet, exercise, and sleep. More often, prescriptions will be written for some sort of professional counseling and/or mild antidepressants. Some people experience a dramatic lifting of depression within days or weeks; others require a longer period of time before any relief is realized. Although treatments don't work for everyone and depression sometimes persists despite therapy, you can't know if treatment will or won't help until you try. New treatments for depression are becoming available every year.

Let your doctors know you might be depressed. Accept help if you are depressed. Doing so is like removing a twenty-pound backpack before hiking up a hill; i.e., you still have a climb ahead of you, but it will be easier and less painful.

What if I feel angry?

Anger is another common, normal reaction to a cancer diagnosis. You may have justified anger about the reaction of certain people to your illness, or some aspect of your medical care. The object of your ire may be more abstract, such as outrage at the unfairness of life. Anger can hurt or help you depending upon what you do with it.

Bottled-up anger drains energy and can interfere with your important relationships, such as those with your physicians, family, friends, or coworkers. You are the one who benefits most from a trusting and congenial alliance with the people who care for and about you. It is in your best interest to find healthy ways to work through anger that keeps you from getting good care or relating to loved ones. Sharing your angry thoughts and feelings with an understanding friend, family member, or counselor may help dissolve your fury. Writing can be a useful tool for venting negative emotions. Nonverbal expression—such as music, art, or exercise—may help, too.

Anger helps you if it motivates you in positive ways. Some survivors who are angry about their illness or prognosis feel empowered and use the energy of their anger to obtain second and third opinions, make wise decisions with their physicians, and do everything possible to help the treatments work as well as possible.

What if I feel anxious?

A feeling of apprehension, worry, uneasiness, or dread is a normal response to a threatening situation. It is normal and expected for you to feel some anxiety about your health, life, and future. For many, anxiety is highest soon after the diagnosis and rises again just before checkups, at the end of treatment, or at other times of increasing uncertainty. Anxiety also can be caused or exacerbated by medical conditions such as hyperthyroidism (high thyroid levels) or sleep deprivation, or by medications such as steroids.

Anxiety is not all bad: It often helps motivate you to purposeful action. However, after your cancer diagnosis, anxiety also can interfere with your ability to get good medical care or tend to your responsibilities. It can disturb your rest and become persistent and/or excessive. Let your health-care team know if you feel anxious and how the anxiety is affecting you. For instance, inform them if you are having trouble sleeping, eating, going for treatments, relating to your family, driving (for fear of an accident), or anything else that might be related to your current level of anxiety.

You don't have to handle a new diagnosis "calmly" to handle it "well." Most people don't remain calm at first. When you are getting good care, and expressing and using your emotions (whatever they might be) to move forward, you are handling it well.

What can be done for anxiety?

Your anxiety may lessen or disappear after you

- acknowledge and talk about your anxiety with loved ones or a professional counselor;

- have your doctors adjust your medications that may be causing or contributing to it;
- get a few good nights' sleep;
- take a short course of mild antianxiety medication (**anxiolytics**);
- learn self-relaxation techniques.

You may simply need a few days or weeks to adjust to the changes. If your anxiety is severe or persistent despite the above measures, you may need more intensive counseling and/or stronger medications.

What if I keep worrying that I made the wrong treatment choice?

Once you have begun a chosen course of treatment, don't second-guess yourself. Since you can't turn the clock back, time and energy spent second-guessing your decision is futile. In most cases, it is best to continue a course of treatment once started, unless complications arise or it becomes clear that your cancer isn't responding. Try to nourish hope and put all your energy into helping the current treatment work.

Once you've made your treatment choice with your physicians, don't look back.

What if I feel that I have become a hypochondriac, worrying about every little ache and pain?

A hypochondriac is someone who suffers from imaginary illnesses or problems. We use the term loosely to apply to anyone who seems overly concerned about his or her health. After learning that you have cancer, you are entitled to be attentive to your body and anxious about new symptoms. It is adaptive and healthy (and *not* hypochondriacal) to be tuned in to your body's signals, especially when you are going through treatment. Real, ongoing physical reactions occur in your body throughout the treatment period. When your body senses something different, you may feel anxious; this is one way that your body brings the physical change to your attention. Since it's easier to ignore a symptom that doesn't make you anxious, anxiety is your friend when it encourages you to get help for a problem.

In chapter 3, some guidelines are presented for when to call your doctors and nurses about a symptom. Two helpful questions are "Am I worried?" and "Am I spending any energy trying not to be concerned?" If the answer to either question is "yes," call your doctor's office and get some professional advice.

Anxiety about a new symptom helps you by bringing potential problems to your attention. Anxiety hurts you when it keeps you from getting good care or living your life.

What if I have a false alarm?

Celebrate the great news! False alarms are an expected part of survivorship. If you knew that a symptom was going to turn out to be a false alarm, you wouldn't have needed to go to the doctor. If your doctors knew it was going to be a false alarm, they wouldn't have needed to examine you or run the tests. You have no reason to feel embarrassed and every reason to feel relieved.

What can I do to feel less anxious about my health?

Once you have brought the symptom or problem to the attention of your doctors, the anxiety is no longer serving a useful function. The following steps may help you to feel less anxious:

- Learn what to expect at each stage of treatment.
- Be informed about your follow-ups.
- Know the signs and symptoms for which you should call or visit your doctor.
- Be in tune with your body, learning to recognize when something is a signal to you that medical attention is needed.
- Be willing to call your doctor's office when you or your family suspects that something is wrong.

Anxiety is a treatable symptom, like nausea or pain. Free-floating anxiety is a drain on your energies and needs intervention. Appropriate counseling and/or safe antianxiety medications can quiet the anxiety.

What if I *don't* feel especially emotional?

Finding out that you have cancer elicits some combination of strong emotions for most people. However, you may feel that you are able to take the news in stride. It may be that you have detached yourself from the situation, doing what you need to do to take care of the problem as if it were happening to someone else. This is a very adaptive coping tool, called dissociation, that some people use without even realizing it. With time, usually days or weeks (but sometimes months or years), the detachment breaks down and the emotional impact of the diagnosis hits home.

Some people truly are able to take crises and traumas in stride with only a little emotional distress. Past experience with major crises, a deep inner understanding and acceptance of the fragility of life, or a singularly unflappable personality style may enable these individuals to sail through stormy seas with little show of emotion.

Staying calm is not better or worse, or right or wrong. What matters is whether you are honest with yourself and others. If you are distressed but trying hard to appear calm, you will use a lot of energy denying normal, genuine feelings. If you really are unruffled, you will create problems by thinking that there is something wrong with the way you are reacting. Be truthful to yourself and others.

What if I feel that I have no control over my life?

A cancer diagnosis causes many people to feel a sense of loss of control over their world. You may feel like you can't control your health, future, or even mundane day-to-day activities. This sense of loss of control can be exaggerated when you are exhausted, in pain, grieving, confused, or dealing with new physical limitations, such as immobility or an inability to control your bladder or bowels.

Control over your world is an illusion. Although you could *affect* your health, job prospects, and family interactions before your cancer diagnosis, you never had complete *control*. You were always at risk of some illness or accident, unexpected problems at work, or family upsets.

Cancer did not cause the lack of control over your world; it revealed it.

How can I regain a sense of control over my world?

Try to focus on the things over which you can maintain control. Sometimes this is a matter of perception. Going for treatments can be seen as a loss of control: "I can't choose what I do today because I have to go for treatment." Or it can be perceived as an activity reflecting great control: "Today, I am choosing to get treatment that will help me get better."

Some practical steps for regaining a sense of control include:

- Draw reasonable limits around what you try to accomplish in a day (or morning, or hour).
- Take satisfaction in what you can get done, even if this is simply getting your cancer treatment, eating, exercising, and resting well.
- Tend to the little things that cause upheaval if neglected.

Sometimes the best short-term solution for a day that feels totally out of control is to go to bed and start again the next morning!

What if I feel like I have no choice about what happens to me?

You always have choices. Granted, you may not have all the choices you want. You can't choose not to have cancer, and you can't choose a painless, easy treatment that guarantees a cure. But you have infinite opportunities within the limited realistic choices. You can choose the best treatment course for you. You can choose your level of understanding and involvement in your care, your relationship with your health-care team, your diet, your support people, your level of hope, and your attitude. Learn about all the realistic choices for every aspect of your well-being, focus on the choices, and then act on them wisely.

What if I just want things to be back to normal?

During treatment, few people can get things back to the way they were before the diagnosis. Too much has changed, and further changes may be on the horizon. In many ways, life is harder and more complicated during cancer treatment. In addition to all life's usual ups and downs, and big and little stresses, you are juggling the extra demands of treatments. The ripple effect can cause disruption in all spheres of your life. Although you can't go back to your old normal life, by learning about what is happening to you and those around you during treatment, you can make choices that help you to create a "new normal" that is healing, meaningful, and even joyful.

Why me?

People who learn that they have cancer often ask, "Why me?" This is a deeply philosophical question, the answer to which touches on your beliefs about life and God. One or more of the following thoughts may help appease this question for you, at least for now:

Unless you had no chance of developing this type of cancer, your illness is in keeping with the probability. If you had a one in a million chance of getting cancer, it was unlikely that you would get it, *but it was a real possibility.* In America, one in three women will develop cancer at some time in their lives; for men, the figure has become one in two. Cancer is such a common disease that millions of people just like you get it. You are not alone.

When cancer is diagnosed, even well-adjusted, mature people can find themselves having thoughts such as "If this bad thing is happening to me, then I must have been bad and cancer is my punishment." This erroneous belief arises from the mistaken application of our society's ethic about blame and punishment. Society deems that people who do something wrong should be punished and should suffer. Wrongdoing → punishment → suffering. However, the reverse does *not* follow; i.e., that if someone is suffering, she or he is being punished for wrongdoing. Since nobody is perfect, everyone can look back with regret or shame at things said or done, thus fueling the notion that they deserved the illness. Usually, this unfounded belief works at a subconscious level.

Another force may contribute to the sense that you deserve your illness: other people's comments about the cause of your disease. They may casually remark about your smoking or drinking, the power lines near your home, your busy work schedule, or your unhealthy diet. You may be left with the generalized feeling that you must have done *something* wrong to cause or deserve your cancer.

Often the comments of friends, family, or strangers are not intended to blame you but to calm *their* fear of becoming ill themselves. If they can point to something you did wrong to cause your cancer, then they can remain safe from cancer by avoiding the bad behavior, whatever it may be. Of course, nobody is immune to illness or death; people just like to think they are.

Many people take solace from the "Why me?" question by asking the corollary question, "Why *not* me?" For many, this is all that is needed to let go of the negative emotions associated with feeling singled out for bad fortune.

Thinking about "Why me?" can make you feel guilty, angry, overwhelmed, helpless, or isolated. Friends, family, clergy, and counselors can help you deal with this question more fully later on. Right now, a more practical and useful question is "What can I do about my situation now?"

The human condition involves pain, loss, and death. Try asking, "Why not me?"

What about my spiritual faith?

A cancer diagnosis challenges your spiritual faith. The effect can vary widely, precipitating intense fear or providing incredible calm. Your faith may fluctuate from day to day, leaving you feeling confused, angry, or lonely. In facing your mortality, especially if for the first time in a meaningful way, you put your spiritual beliefs to the test. A cancer diagnosis often prompts patients to ask the big questions such as, "What is the meaning of life?" "What is the meaning of *my* life?" "Do I believe in God?" "Where is God in my time of trouble?" In trying to answer these questions with the new perspective offered by your illness, you can understand and ultimately find comfort in whatever you believe.

You may find yourself questioning things that you thought you were sure about, or thinking about things you'd never let yourself think about before. Try to see the uncertainty accompanying your diagnosis as an opportunity to discover or confirm what you believe. The process of exploring your faith may be difficult, painful, or frightening. Share your thoughts and feelings with understanding friends, family, clergy, or counselors. Tending to your spiritual self is healing.

How should I feel if something I did may have caused the cancer or allowed it to get as far as it did?

If you did something in the past that may have contributed to your current cancer situation, such as smoking cigarettes or delaying a mammogram, it is understandable if you feel guilty about getting sick. Guilt is good when it helps you to do the right thing, not when you torment yourself. Focusing on what you should have done, or could have done, is destructive, wasted energy. Blaming yourself helps no one else and hurts you. You can't change the past. Chances are you downplayed, denied, or didn't appreciate the risks of your behavior before you were diagnosed with cancer. Ask yourself if you smoked cigarettes or skipped your annual mammogram or rectal exam *with the intent of* getting sick and causing your family distress. If the answer is "no," forgive yourself for being human and imperfect. Your mind allowed you to believe that you could escape harm. This is similar to the mind-set that allows millions of people to drive too fast or without seat belts, saying to themselves, "I know that car accidents kill and maim every day, but it won't happen to me."

Forgive yourself for anything in the past that may have contributed to your illness.

What is denial?

Technically speaking, denial is an abnormal refusal to accept the truth. In this book, the word "denial" will be used loosely, as it is by most nonpsychiatrists, to mean anything from unhealthy denial of the truth to healthy repression of painful truths.

Is denial a good thing?

Denial is an adaptive tool that allows us to function in a world marked by uncertainties and dangers. Emotionally healthy people use denial every day. If people thought about all the bad things that could happen every time they drove a car, ate in a restaurant, or allowed their children to ride bicycles, they would be immobilized by fear and anxiety. It is healthy and normal to use appropriate denial *as long as our behavior is responsible.*

While you are going through cancer treatments and doing well, denying the possibility of treatment related complications or the possibility of needing more treatment after completing your current course are examples of healthy, adaptive repression that helps you get through. However, if you deny that you have cancer, or deny symptoms or problems, and consequently don't take advantage of effective treatments, you are risking your health and your life. If you deny that you are having a hard time emotionally, socially, spiritually, or financially when, in fact, things are rocky, and if you turn down help from others, you are denying yourself services and opportunities for improved well-being and growth. This kind of denial is not helpful.

Right now, you may be imagining all the possible horrible things that could happen. If so, you have temporarily lost your ability for healthy denial. Usually, your wall of denial will be rebuilt over time, although it may never be as solid as it was before your diagnosis. If your ability to push worrisome thoughts or fears out of your mind does not improve over time, you can learn techniques to help you regain the ability to deny. Healthy denial (repression) helps you through frightening times.

Denial is bad when it keeps you from seeking effective treatment or assistance.
Denial is good when it helps you get good care and live as fully as possible.

What about counseling?

Counseling is one way to help you deal with any stress or challenge, be it a new job, rocky marriage, or serious illness. Good counselors bring experience, objectivity, and caring to your personal trials and tribulations. Unlike friends or family, professional counselors can't be hurt by anything you think, say, or do, so the focus is always on helping *you* deal with *your* challenges. Counseling helps you to

- clarify the practical problems and establish a foundation for overcoming them;
- clarify the emotional concerns and establish a foundation for dealing with them in healthy ways;
- work through the obstacles to realistic solutions;
- recognize problems that can't be fixed and learn to adjust to them;
- feel less alone in your pain and struggles.

How do I know if I need professional counseling?

Many people who have weathered life's ups and downs in the past without difficulty, and who are reacting normally to their new cancer diagnosis, benefit from interaction with a professional counselor. Counseling may shorten the time you need to adjust and can help make your transitions easier. Don't hesitate to have your oncologist refer you to a trained therapist if you are feeling overwhelmed, afraid, anxious, depressed, or if you are having difficulty concentrating, relating to others, or fulfilling your responsibilities.

You don't have to be in a crisis or emotionally unstable to benefit from counseling. Athletes improve their athletic performance by working with trainers who help them understand and use their emotions to enhance their physical performance. In a similar way, well-adjusted people who are dealing with the expected challenges of cancer can benefit from "trainers" called counselers.

Right now, your body demands extra energy for physical healing. Don't spend weeks or months wasting precious energy dealing with difficult emotions and thoughts without help if you don't have to. Consider seeing a counselor sooner rather than later if any of the following circumstances persist:

- You feel unable to communicate with your family or friends.
- You are having difficulty eating or sleeping, and your medical evaluation doesn't provide an explanation.
- You feel overwhelmed.
- You feel that unresolved problems unrelated to your cancer have surfaced or intensified and are distressing. Energy directed toward these other problems is unavailable for making wise treatment decisions and adjusting to treatment.

Even if everything is going as smoothly as possible, you may wish to pursue counseling to help you

- participate effectively in your treatments;
- maximize the emotional or spiritual growth that can come from this experience.

THE MIND-BODY CONNECTION

Does the mind affect the body?

Yes. Your mind affects your body. Stop for a moment and picture in your mind a juicy lemon being cut in half. Now imagine yourself licking the cut surface. I suspect your salivary glands are tingling and you have a burst of saliva in your mouth even though you are simply thinking of the lemon. If you hear a door slam behind you, your heart may race. If you throw a ball, you'll have a better chance of hitting your target if your mind is focused.

Not only does your mind affect your body; your body also affects your mind. If you haven't slept in two days, your thinking may be cloudy. If you have a high fever, you may experience hallucinations. If you suffer from chronic pain, you may feel depressed.

What about the stories of people using their minds to cure cancer?

There is NO evidence that people with cancer can "think" or "will" themselves well again without also taking effective anticancer treatments.

The human body is programmed to try to heal itself whenever it becomes injured or sick. The mind plays an important role in this self-healing. Expecting and wanting to get better seem to help people recover. Patients with terminal diseases who expect to die seem to do worse or die more quickly than those who want to recover. However, the mind only *affects* the body; it does not *control* the body. Some patients receive excellent care and focus the power of their minds against their cancer yet still succumb to disease that couldn't be controlled with the best of treatment and attitude. And other patients give up all hope and make no apparent effort to survive other than receiving effective treatments to please family members, yet they enjoy uneventful recoveries and live long lives.

The mind affects the body; it does not control the body.

How important is my will to live?

Your will to live is one aspect of the power of your mind that plays a role in how well you do during and after treatment. Although, by itself, a strong will to live doesn't guarantee survival, it may

- encourage you to comply with treatments, eat well, be more active, nourish your relationships with others, grow spiritually;
- help you feel better physically, emotionally, and spiritually;
- cause physical changes that improve your chance of cure or long life.

What is a positive attitude?

A positive attitude is one that helps you positively. For Healthy Survivors, a positive attitude helps you get good care and live as fully as possible within the constraints of your illness. The key is having a foundation of hope—a belief that you can affect your outcome and quality of life in positive ways.

What is the difference between optimism and a positive attitude?

Optimism means you expect a good outcome. A positive attitude means that you are hopeful that you can affect your outcome in

positive ways, not that you are positive (i.e., sure) that you are
going to have a good outcome. Given that you don't have any
guarantees in life, to be 100 percent confident of a good outcome
is unrealistic for most people. If you try to be completely sure of
a good outcome, you deny yourself the expression of normal,
healthy fear, grief, and anxiety. And, it takes extra energy to
appear optimistic or happy on days that are really bad because of
illness or social stresses. A positive attitude includes times of fear-
fulness, sadness, anger, hopelessness, and other unpleasant (and
normal) emotions and thoughts.

**A positive attitude is one that helps you get good care, find
and nourish hope, and live your life as fully as possible,
today.**

How important is a positive attitude?

As defined above, a positive attitude may help your recovery.
Certainly, it will improve your ongoing quality of life.

What if people are urging me to be happy?

You have plenty of reasons to feel unhappy, and it's okay to feel so,
as long as you don't get stuck feeling this way. Trying to ignore
real problems and genuine feelings in the name of keeping a positive attitude makes it harder (or impossible) to integrate real experiences into your life so you can move forward. Any attitude that
denies your feelings can be more stressful to your system than
working through the painful, embarrassing, or shameful thoughts
and emotions that accompany life's challenges.

Is there a "best" attitude for me?

The best attitude is whatever works well for you *at the time.* Open
your mind to different outlooks, approaches, and styles for coping with the stresses and uncertainties of cancer treatment. Try
out new ideas that may work for you; reject those that can't possibly help. Be flexible. Be honest with yourself. Since your situation is dynamic, it follows that a healthy attitude is dynamic, too.
What works well today may not work tomorrow; what didn't

work yesterday may work today. Reconsider approaches that you rejected in the past.

A healthy attitude changes as you and your circumstances change.

Do I need to control the stress in my life if I want to get well?

No. Stress plays a role in health and illness. The idea that you may improve your chance for recovery with healthy stress *management* is not a new concept, and is accepted as truth by most lay and professional people. The dangerous twist added in many discussions of stress (in books and articles, on talk shows, and so on) is that you must *control* all stress to get well and stay well. You can't control the world around you. And you can't avoid stress, especially during cancer treatment. For most people, having cancer and undergoing chemotherapy or radiation, itself, is very stressful. And the little and big bumps in life don't stop just because you're sick: Chores need to be done, children squabble, monthly bills await, and friends and family suffer their own tragedies. Your fate is not doomed if you grieve the loss of a loved one, struggle with family problems, or lose your job. Normal life carries pain, loss, worry, and good and bad stresses. Protecting yourself from hard times isolates you physically and emotionally from your world. The whole reason for going through treatment is to live your life, not to hide from it. Facing the hard times, with support if necessary, can free you to deal with your treatments and still enjoy the good things in your life.

What can I do to decrease my stress level during treatment?

Managing life's stress may help your recovery. At the very least, it will make you feel better. Think about stress management in a realistic way that fits your personality and preferred lifestyle. There is no one right way to manage stress. What causes unpleasant stress for one person may be invigorating to another (such as deadlines at work or exercising at the gym). What is a relaxing activity for one (such as meditating) may be nerve-wracking for another. What is an avoidable issue for some (such as problems with coworkers or relatives) is inescapable for others.

Examine the various stresses in your life and figure out which ones are *positive* (i.e., they help you feel energized or refreshed) and which ones are *negative* (i.e., they drain your reserves). Note that certain activities that were rejuvenating before your illness—such as your exercise routine or work schedule—may need to be modified under the current circumstances in order to continue to be helpful.

Look at the various stresses and determine which ones you have a choice about during treatment. You may have to deal with the demands of raising your own children and/or caring for a chronically ill parent, working for a boss who is a reincarnation of Atilla the Hun, or stretching an inadequate income. For unavoidable problems, get help learning how to

- accept the necessary stress;
- minimize the associated stress;
- deal with your feelings in healthy ways.

When you do have choices, figure out what is best for you. Sometimes the hardest step is recognizing that, indeed, you do have choices about many of life's pressures. For the time of your treatments:

- Are there any chores that can be delegated or neglected? It may help if, over the next few months, you lower your standards for a clean house, cut down on volunteer work, let someone else help care for a sick parent, or take advantage of convenience foods or services.
- Are there problems that you can decide to take care of later? Can some repair jobs wait? Can an entanglement with a neighbor be let go for now?
- Are there decisions that can be postponed?

Don't make the common mistake of thinking you don't have any choices. Sometimes the hardest step is recognizing that, indeed, you do have choices about many of life's pressures. If you feel stressed, a one-time consultation with a social worker or other counselor may help you see some choices you didn't know you had.

What if I worry about not doing enough to have a healthy attitude or manage my stress?

There are many possible explanations for why you may worry about your attitude or stress level, even after taking steps to find a healthy balance. For one thing, from the day of diagnosis on, you may be inundated with prescriptions for attitudes and stress-management programs from family, friends, and even strangers. These well-intentioned words of advice may have detrimental effects. If you dismiss others' advice because you don't believe in, for example, the anticancer effect of visualizing your chemo as Pacmen eating your cancer cells, you may feel worried or guilty about not doing everything possible to regain your health. Strain can arise between you and your friends and loved ones if you seem to be rejecting their suggestions. Noncommittal following of others' advice also can cause you to feel hypocritical (and stressed).

Another source of discomfort may be that you wish to make changes in your life but find them hard to enact right now. Going through times of transition and forming new habits is stressful, even when the changes are for the better. Don't feel the need to fix everything or anything right now. You will have a better idea of what you want to change, and in what order and how, after you've made a treatment decision and are adjusting to all the changes.

If you have fleeting or lingering self-doubts about your decision to spurn a daily meditation program or avoid visits with relatives who upset you, it may be because you've made an unwise choice. More likely, you have put healthy, rational decisions into action but are having a hard time accepting your limits and/or the negative fallout accompanying a positive move. The best you can do is the best you can do. Focus on the healthy choices you've made, and embrace them so you can live the life you have.

What is a "cancer personality"?

The notion of a cancer personality—a type of person who is more likely to get cancer because of his or her personality—is silly. All different types of people get cancer: placid and excitable people, shy and brazen people, missionaries and gangsters, and innocent babies. Millions of people with the supposed cancer personality don't get cancer. Your personality did not cause your cancer.

It is interesting to look back in history at our ancestors' explanations for illnesses that are now well-defined. For example, before the infection-causing organism responsible for tuberculosis was discovered, people hypothesized about a "tuberculosis personality." When the responsible microbe was discovered, the idea of a "tuberculosis personality" vanished.

What if I feel hopeless?

Hope is the belief that something you *want* to happen *can* happen. Healthy Survivors nourish a particular hope: the belief that they can do something to help their situation. Hope is a dynamic, complex phenomenon that is affected by many factors. All other things being equal, it is harder to feel hopeful if

- the statistics for your type of cancer are unfavorable;
- you are in pain or feel sick;
- you've had bad experiences with similar challenges;
- you have an innate tendency toward pessimism;
- your doctors and nurses, friends and family convey hopelessness about your situation.

The ancient Roman philosopher Cicero said, "While there's life, there's hope." Unless you are near death at this moment without any treatment options, you can find and nourish hope of improvement. Besides hoping for remission and cure, you can hope for relief from pain, an improved sense of well-being, the repair of a relationship, another celebration, or one more kiss.

There is always hope. Find and nourish hope.

How can I nourish hope?

Use life-enhancing language. You are a cancer survivor, not a cancer victim. Your treatments are not toxic poisons but powerful tonics aimed at restoring your health.

Talk with other survivors. Meeting another person who was in a similar cancer situation and is now doing well puts a name and face to the idea that you can land on the good side of the statistics and go on to live a full and healthy life.

Avoid being with people who are hopeless and who insist on sharing their pessimistic perspectives.

Find ways that your situation is unique or different from the group of patients with your prognosis. If you do this, your prognosis may no longer feel like a verdict. For example, if you are younger or older than the average patient with your type of cancer, you may do better. So, too, you may do better if you are athletic, or if you have relatives with the same cancer who did well, or if you have always eaten a healthful diet, or if there is something else that makes you special.

Find ways that you can bolster your body, such as with sound nutrition and doctor-approved physical activity. Tend to your emotional and spiritual needs, too, with activities that are calming, satisfying, and enriching. For some, that may be working in a garden or painting; for others, it may be playing basketball or participating in a book club, singing in a choir or studying the psalms.

Make plans for the future such as enjoying a lunch date tomorrow, playing a game of checkers next week, listening to a concert next month, or attending a graduation in two years. If making plans for years, months, or weeks from now causes you to feel anxious, make plans only for a time frame within which you are comfortable.

Voice your fears, either alone in the shower or in a quiet park or, preferably, in the company of caring friends, family, a support group, or a professional counselor or clergyperson. Write them down on a piece of paper or think through them in prayer. Naming and sharing fears often helps tame them.

What if I am having negative thoughts or dreams?

Negative thoughts and dreams—such as dreams of getting bad news or having loved ones abandon you—are normal and expected. As you adjust to the reality of having a life-threatening illness, your mind may play with all the possible scenarios you fear, including complications and death. These thoughts and nightmares do not reflect what you believe will happen or want to happen *unless you interpret them that way.*

Can negative thoughts cause my condition to get worse?

No. Negative thoughts are a normal part of the cancer experience. If pessimistic thoughts caused cancer to grow, nobody would survive cancer. They are harmful if you choose to replay them over and over in your mind, and thus stir up the associated emotions. They are dangerous if you interpret them to mean that your fate is sealed, causing you to give up on treatments and measures that offer you realistic hope for recovery. Negative thoughts are helpful if they encourage you to talk about the things that frighten or upset you.

Negative thoughts can coexist with a deep faith in a complete recovery.

What can I do about my negative thoughts and dreams?

See your negative thoughts and dreams as signals for topics that need to be discussed. When you have bothersome thoughts or nightmares, talk about them with someone who understands, work through the problems or feelings that caused them, and then let the negative thoughts go. Remind yourself that they are a normal part of dealing with serious illness and that they in no way foretell your future. If you tend to dwell on negative thoughts, especially to the exclusion of more positive thoughts, you may be depressed or genuinely feel hopeless and you may benefit from psychological or spiritual counseling.

Will being hopeful make things worse if the outcome is not good?

No. Complications and poor outcomes are distressing whether you expect them or not. Everyone must find his or her own unique comfort zone for hope. Recognizing the possibility of a poor outcome while hoping for a good one is usually a helpful approach no matter what the ultimate outcome. Try to gear your level of hope to what maximizes your quality of life *now* and not to what you think will make it easier to receive bad or good news in the future.

How can I accept the scary facts about my disease and still be hopeful?

Your mind is able to accept the likelihood of a bad outcome while, at the same time, maintaining hope for an unexpectedly good outcome. Some call this "hopeful acceptance," or "hope without expectations." The balance between acceptance and hope will shift as your circumstances fluctuate. For example, you can accept that most people who receive your type of chemotherapy will lose their hair. Based on this acceptance, you may go ahead and arrange for a wig. But until your hair actually falls out, you can have realistic hope that you will be one of the few who don't lose their hair. This hope will fade quickly and appropriately if your hair starts to fall out. As another example, you can accept the fact that your type of cancer tends to recur yet still be hopeful that you are one of the few who are cured with a single round of treatment.

FAMILY CONCERNS

Do I have to tell my family?

Yes, in most cases. Ask yourself, "Would I want to be informed if one of my family members was diagnosed with this cancer?" Despite the emotional pain it causes, the best course of action is usually to share the news of your diagnosis as well as the ups and downs of treatment. Close relatives will sense that something is wrong, even without your saying anything, and may imagine possibilities that are far worse than the truth. Also, it takes more energy for you to maintain a lie than to handle the fallout of sharing the diagnosis. When you include your family in the crisis, they can help you to

- get good medical care;
- take care of daily responsibilities;
- endure the emotional highs and lows of evaluation and treatment;
- find and nourish hope.

In exceptional circumstances, you may sense that it would be unwise to reveal your diagnosis to a family member who is unstable, physically or mentally. The best course of action depends on the specifics of their situation, your relationship with them, and your medical condition and prognosis. It may help to get advice from a neutral party such as a social worker.

What if some of my family members have become worried about getting cancer themselves?

It is understandable that relatives may become more conscious of any symptoms they may have or simply become worried that they, too, will develop cancer. After all, if you could get cancer, then they could. At the same time, family members may hesitate to take care of their own health needs, reasoning, "I don't want to add any more problems right now. I'll take care of it when you're better." When a relative has any symptoms or is at high risk for cancer, it is best for everyone if he or she gets it checked out now by a doctor. If there is a problem, it can be addressed in a timely manner. If there is not a problem, the reassurance will relieve everyone.

What about sex?

It is common for people's interest in sex to diminish or disappear after they are first diagnosed with cancer. Sexual desire and sexual function can be affected by:

- Physical problems or changes
- Pain
- Some cancer treatments
- Medications
- Stress
- Anxiety
- Depression
- Fatigue

Volumes have been written about the effects of cancer and treatment on sexual function and sexual satisfaction. Doctors, nurses, counselors, and support groups are trained to guide you through this transition. If you have questions, concerns, anxieties, or problems, let your doctor know. Your sexuality is a part of your normal functioning, just like your eating, sleeping, and breathing. By sharing your questions and problems with your doctors and nurses, you can decrease the chance of unnecessary restrictions and limitations, or future problems with sexuality. Whereas sexual desire may be diminished, your need for intimacy may be increased. Being close, hugging, and talking privately are important ways to combat loneliness and isolation. It is important for you and for those who care about you to maintain contact.

Why are things strained with some of my family members?

Even under ideal circumstances, being diagnosed with cancer causes strain in family relationships. This is because your entire family is in a period of transition, with everyone experiencing

- a host of strong emotions;
- changes in roles and responsibilities;
- disrupted routines;
- uncertainty about your well-being, and their own well-being;
- uncertainty about the future (home, work, finances).

For the first time in their lives, your loved ones may be unsure of what to do or say to help you. They may keep their own worries to themselves for fear of burdening you, thus widening the communication gap.

Relationships that were shaky before your diagnosis may be further strained by the demands of your illness. Oftentimes, difficult relationships just get worse under the added stress, at least temporarily. Hopefully, these people can rise to the occasion, and your cancer will catalyze healing and strengthening of relationships.

What if I find my family's advice annoying or intrusive?

It is important to understand what may be motivating your family to voice their beliefs about your illness and prescriptions for your recovery, and why receiving advice from them may be difficult for you. Possibilities to consider include:

- They love you and believe their advice can help you.
- Heightened emotions may cause them to lose sight of their usual boundaries for offering advice.
- They are tired and overstressed from juggling the demands of their usual responsibilities while trying to help you.
- Tension is due to the flare-up of past problems in the setting of your illness. Just when they need to be pulling together, families may play out old power struggles without realizing it.
- You may be overwhelmed by your medical problems; *any* advice seems like too much.
- Your sense of self may be threatened by the illness; advice from others furthers this loss of self-esteem.

This is an especially difficult time for you to deal with family problems, more stress, or more loss. Your doctor or nurse or a social worker can refer you to someone trained in family problems, preferably someone experienced in illness-related family stress.

What about the well partner?

When you get sick, your well partner dons many hats: companion, cheerleader, caregiver, and communicator for your friends and family, to name just a few. For many well partners, new roles and responsibilities fall on their shoulders in addition to their usual ones. Their self-esteem may be damaged by their sense of powerlessness to protect you from the necessary risks and discomforts of your illness. Some of their emotions mirror yours; others are unique.

In certain ways, it is harder to be the well partner. As the patient, *you can act* and get treatment. Everyone expects you, the patient, to have special needs; they try to anticipate and tend to them. While everyone is focused on your needs, your partner has new and increased needs, too. Everyone suffers when your partner's needs go unnoticed or are not met.

How can I help my partner?

A few simple steps may help to prevent or minimize problems for the well partner:

- Keep the communication open and *two*-way as much as possible.
- Encourage breaks from the seriousness and responsibilities of your illness.
- Get help with chores.
- Take advantage of the books, newsletters, reputable Web sites, and support services/groups for caregivers.

Should I tell my children that I have cancer?

Yes. The cancer may have happened to you, but the cancer experience is happening to your entire family. Open communication in an atmosphere of love and realistic hope is vital to your children's healthy adjustment to your illness. Even if you never say a word, they sense that something is going on. They are trying to understand what is happening. Your being candid with them opens the opportunity to lead them to a healthy understanding of your illness, and to adaptive coping skills. If you try to keep your illness a secret in an attempt to protect your children, their imaginations may lead them to conclusions and fears that are much worse than the real situation, and to coping skills that are maladaptive.

A conspiracy of silence forces your children to keep their fears, insecurities, and questions to themselves. Also, it is a lot more work *for you* to maintain a lie than to deal with the fallout of sharing the truth. Open communication allows you to be their ally in dealing with any hard times that may lie ahead.

The greatest gift you can give your children is not protection from the world but the confidence and tools to cope and grow through life's challenges.

What do my children need?

Children have three fundamental needs:

- Ongoing satisfaction of their basic physical and emotional needs (such as food, shelter, and love)
- An understanding *on their level* of what is happening in *their*

world (such as why Dad is in the hospital, why Mom is bald, or why Mom and Dad are crying behind closed doors)
- Reassurance that they will be cared for no matter what happens (such as who will drive them to school or soccer, and who will tuck them into bed at night)

In particular, children whose parent has cancer need

- information that is truthful and clear;
- to feel involved and important;
- reassurance that other caring adults will step in for a parent who is unavailable due to illness;
- encouragement to maintain their own interests and activities;
- to feel it is okay to have their own thoughts and feelings;
- to have regular contact with caring adults with whom it is safe to express their own thoughts and feelings.

Who should break the news of my diagnosis to my children?

It's best if the news about your diagnosis, as well as about setbacks or complications, is delivered by you or your spouse, provided you can handle it. Crying and showing emotions is appropriate and acceptable. Your children will learn that this is a difficult time for you, and that it's normal to be upset for a while. Be direct so they do not misinterpret what they are seeing: "I am crying because I am sad that I am sick, and nervous about some of the changes. But I will tell you what you need to know, and help you adjust."

If you are uncontrollably upset, your children may feel afraid and insecure no matter how perfect your choice of words. When this is the case, it is better for another adult who is close to the children—such as the other parent, a grandparent, or close family friend—to talk with them. If your illness or the need to travel for second opinions keeps you from your children, consider having a trusted friend or relative break the news and explain why you couldn't do it yourself. *Your top priority is doing everything possible to get well.*

What are the goals of breaking the news to my children?

- To provide enough facts to allay their immediate fears
- To reassure them that they will be kept informed and be well taken care of
- To prepare them for what is coming next

How do I break the news?

Find a quiet place where you can hold them and not be interrupted. *Tell them that you have cancer, the name of your cancer, and that you are going to be treated.* It is much better to tell them yourself than risk their overhearing it in your conversations with others, or hearing it for the first time from someone else who may paint an unfounded gloomy picture. By hearing it from you, they know that they can trust you to tell them the truth about what is going on.

Tell them that cancer is a disease that can be treated. Children can have negative preconceptions about cancer from television, friends' comments, or their interpretation of what is happening around them. If it is expected that you will do well, you need to say this directly.

Explain that cancer is not contagious. They cannot get cancer from you. They did not give the cancer to you. Don't assume that children know this. Explain, too, that they are not responsible for your illness or the outcome. Children often believe that you got cancer because they did something bad, or even just thought something bad. You may need to reinforce this over and over throughout your course of treatment.

Reassure your children, including teenagers, that their needs will be satisfied. It is normal and healthy for children to be anxious and/or angry about what is going to happen *to them.* As upsetting and demanding as your situation may seem to you, you must remember that this crisis is affecting your children's lives, too. If you cannot tend to their needs, ask someone else to be there to provide physical and emotional support. You may save yourself and your children from future problems by ensuring that a caring and capable adult is being responsive to their needs now.

Are my children too young to tell about my cancer?

No. If they are old enough for you to tell them that your leg is in a cast because you broke it, or that you are taking a nap because you are tired, you can and should tell them that you have cancer and need treatment to get well. The specifics of what you say will depend upon each child's age, maturity, past experiences, and level of interest. Certainly, your babies are too young to tell about your cancer. However, cancer treatments often last months; cancer-related family stresses and problems can last even longer. Consequently, sometime during the course of your treatment or recovery, they may get to an age when they need to know about your illness. Since your cancer will no longer be news to you, it would be easy to forget that your little ones were never told directly about your diagnosis or treatment. They will need you to talk with them as you would if you all just found out about your cancer.

It is better to err on the side of telling them too much, too soon than too little, too late. You tell your children "I love you" and "Here's a spoonful of yummy applesauce" long before they can really understand or respond. You can provide words of truth, comfort, and hope before they understand them: "Daddy has cancer and he's taking radiation and medicines to make him better." When they first become able to grasp that you have cancer, they will already possess the beginning tools to deal with it in healthy and hopeful ways.

Will the word "cancer" scare them?

Even though you may feel uncomfortable saying "cancer," using it in front of your children helps make "cancer" just another ordinary word, and not forbidden, scary, or emotionally charged. Naming something that is confusing or terrifying, and calling it by its name, are two powerful ways to gain a sense of control. The word "cancer" usually does not carry the negative connotations for your children that it may for you.

Using the specific name of your disease, such as "sarcoma," "colon cancer," or "lymphoma," helps to distance your disease from those of people with other types of cancer, some of whom may have had bad experiences or outcomes.

Do I have to tell the truth?

Yes. Telling the truth is the *only* way to establish and maintain your children's trust. The way to help protect them from being overwhelmed is not with a lie but with the love and support that surround telling them the truth.

Always tell the truth, couched in love and hopefulness.

What if I just can't bring myself to break the news?

Ask a friend, relative, social worker, or family counselor to meet with you and your children. They can explain the situation for you and establish open communication between you and your children. Usually, it gets easier after one or two meetings, and you can continue the dialogue on your own. If your family needs occasional or ongoing assistance with communication, there are people who can help. It's better to depend on others to help you with this difficult task than to insist on doing it yourself and end up not doing it at all.

Fox Chase Cancer Center has developed an eighteen-minute video that shows parents how to break the news and take those first painful steps toward surviving as a family. *Talking about Your Cancer: a Parent's Guide to Helping Children Cope.* Copies are available for $29.95 each plus $5.00 shipping and handling by calling 215-728-2668 or writing to the Department of Social Work Services at the Fox Chase Cancer Center, 7701 Burholme Avenue, Philadelphia, PA 19111.

Do I have to tell my children everything?

No. *Tell them enough, not everything.* How much is enough is determined by each child's personal need for information. Some children adjust best if given every little detail, down to the milligram doses of your medicines and a play-by-play of how you are feeling (which can be draining for you). Others do better if told only the most rudimentary facts that they need to know. In order to meet each child's specific needs, it may be best to talk to each one individually. The ongoing process of tending to children with different needs is challenging.

In addition, each child's need for information and support likely will vary from time to time, depending on what is happening to you and where they are in their understanding and adjustment. Tell each child what he or she wants and needs to know at the time. Keeping the lines of communication open is the best insurance for making sure they get enough information.

Should I tell my children's pediatrician or teachers about my illness?

Absolutely. Your children's pediatrician, school guidance counselor, and teachers can give you specific guidance about how best to deal with your children. Do not wait for a problem to develop before you seek the input and involvement of these professionals.

In addition to your children's schoolteachers, you might want to talk with their music or dance teachers, sports coaches, and other important adults in their lives. Tell them what is going on, how you are handling it with the children, and how you would like them to deal with your illness when they are relating to your children. In this way, the important adults in your children's lives will interpret your children's behavior and performance in the context of your illness, and can be alert to problems that you may need to address.

In general, it is best if school and extracurricular activities remain places where your children can forget about the troubles at home, and can focus on their studies and friends. You might want to request that teachers do not ask your children about your well-being unless the children bring it up first. Depending upon the chemistry between a particular adult and your child, your kids' teachers or coaches can be valuable confidants for youngsters who are having a hard time. Improve the ability of other adults to help your children by staying in touch with them.

What if my children are more irritable, sleeping poorly, not eating well, or performing poorly at school or at home?

Your children's behavior and performance may slip as they adjust to the news and all the changes. Irritability and backslides ("regression") are often signs of children's stress and increased needs. Youngsters usually regain lost ground and resume their usual eating and sleeping habits when the crisis settles down and a new routine is established. *Continued* problems suggest that they have needs that are not being met adequately. Involve other adults, including your children's pediatrician and teachers, to determine how your children are doing and how you can help them through your illness.

What if my children ask me if I'm going to die?

You can be honest and, at the same time, calm their fears and encourage hopefulness. Your exact answer will be shaped by innumerable factors, including:

- The age and maturity of the child
- What conversations and experiences you've had in the past about death
- The specifics of your medical situation
- Your spiritual beliefs

If your prognosis is good, tell your children something like "Cancer can make some people die, but *most* people with *my type of cancer* get well. I am planning on getting well again. I'll tell you if the cancer is ever getting worse." Don't be afraid to admit to your children that cancer is life-threatening. They will worry less if you tell them so than if you tell a half-truth, avoid the topic, or tell a flat-out lie. Don't forget that they draw their own conclusions based on what you say (or don't say) *and* from signals they are seeing, hearing, and sensing in other, more subtle ways.

If your prognosis is poor but treatment is available, you can answer with something like "Everyone dies, and I'm going to die one day. Many people with this type of cancer don't get better (or get better for a while and then get sick again) and die from the cancer. But a few people do get well again. We are doing everything possible to help me be one of the few who gets all better. I will tell you if the treatments aren't working and the cancer is getting worse. Right now, let's hope for the best."

This answer is a brief introduction to a highly emotional, complex topic. The annotated bibliography in my book *When a Parent Has Cancer: A Guide to Caring for Your Children* (HarperCollins) can refer you to numerous valuable resources for dealing with uncertainty and serious illness with your children.

Tell your children the truth in a hopeful and loving way. Keep the lines of communication open. Reassure your children that they will be cared for no matter what happens.

What if my children get upset when I tell the truth?

Expect your children to get upset! Children get upset when they learn upsetting news. This is a normal, healthy, healing way to begin adjusting to hard times. Their crying or screaming may be painful for you to witness, but it indicates that they understand to some degree what is going on (which is good) and that they are reacting (which is also good). Children often express emotions differently than adults. They may become uncharacteristically withdrawn and quiet, or sassy and rebellious. They may be hysterically upset one moment, and the next moment you'll see them playing as if they didn't have a care in the world. Comfort your children. Give them a safe place to express their emotions, whatever their emotions may be. Reassure them that their negative feelings will lessen with time.

It is a good sign when children feel safe enough to express negative emotions. Help them work through their feelings and find healthy ways to move forward.

Will my children be emotionally scarred by my illness?

Your children will be affected by your illness. Your words, actions, and love will affect whether the overall impact is positive or negative. Factors beyond your control also will influence how your children integrate this experience into their perception of the world. Obviously, a short, smooth course of treatment that results in a parent's complete recovery is less disruptive and traumatic for the children than a long, rocky course that leads to a parent's permanent disability or premature death.

People are the product of all their life experiences—the good and the bad, the pleasant and the miserable, the happy and the sad, the successes and the failures. Sometimes an adult's greatest gifts or strengths arise from childhood experiences with challenge or loss.

Help your children through the crisis of your illness by

- accepting that cancer has become part of your family's life;
- trying to use your cancer as a strengthening force in the life of your family;
- establishing and maintaining open, two-way communication;
- always telling the truth.

Where can I go for more information on handling the twin challenges of cancer and parenting?

The various aspects of raising children (babies, preschoolers, youngsters, teenagers, and young adults) while dealing with cancer are discussed in my book *When a Parent Has Cancer: A Guide to Caring for Your Children* (HarperCollins). This book contains a separate illustrated children's book, *Becky and the Worry Cup,* to share with your children.

SUPPORT GROUPS

What is a support group?

Generally speaking, a support group is any person or group that is willing and able to help you, emotionally or physically. A support group also may refer to an organized group that meets regularly to deal with cancer-related topics. Some cancer support groups include people with any type of cancer who get together to deal with concerns and feelings common to all cancer patients. Other groups are geared toward people with specific cancers (e.g., prostate, breast, lymphoma), specific situations (e.g., children, young adults, or parents with cancer; post-transplant survivors), or specific problems (e.g., ostomy, loss of vocal cords, amputations). Some groups are intended for patients only, others for patients and their family members, and still others include only the family members and caretakers. Some meet for a set period of time (e.g., six weeks); others are open-ended (the group keeps meeting on schedule; people come to as many meetings as they wish). Some provide a forum for lectures and are topic oriented, while others are unstructured so that people can talk about whatever is on their minds at a given session.

Virtual support groups are available on the Internet. The American Cancer Society offers the Cancer Survivors Network that allows you to hear and read about others' experiences, and converse with other suvivors. This service enables you to obtain topic-oriented insights and support in the privacy of your home at a time that is convenient for you. Their Web site is www.acscsn.org.

Do I need to participate in a support group?

If you are physically able, it's a good idea to try participating in a support group at least two or three times. Support groups can:

- Provide practical information from veteran survivors.
- Provide a support network *separate* from family, coworkers, and close friends. This is especially helpful for people who have chosen to minimize the involvement of their established relationships.
- Provide a support network of people who truly understand because they had cancer, too.
- Provide exposure to people who have found ways to live fully despite limitations imposed by their cancer or cancer history.
- Put real faces and names to the general notion that people survive unfavorable odds and recurrent cancer. This will nourish your hope of doing well.
- Provide a place where you may feel more comfortable talking about difficult topics than in a one-on-one conversation with a family member.
- Provide a place where family and friends can learn more about what the experience of surviving cancer is like for you and others, as well as how best to help you and themselves.
- Show you by example how to find humor, opportunity for growth, or meaning in difficult circumstances.
- Provide a place where having cancer is the norm but the focus is not on treatment.
- Provide another safe place to share good and bad times.

Are there any downsides to going to a support group?

Support groups are not for everyone. You may find it frightening or upsetting to see other people who are worse off than you, or to hear someone who has a pessimistic attitude or depressing personality. Also, the quality of each support group varies (even each meeting of the same group) depending upon the theme, the leaders, and the individuals who participate. In general, a group with a trained facilitator such as a social worker or oncology nurse avoids some of the problems that can occur when participants tend toward counterproductive discussion and behavior. The only way to know if a support group will be beneficial to you or your family is to try one for a few sessions. Warning: Do not attend a support group that claims to be a substitute for medical care.

How do I find out about the support groups available to me?

You can find out about support groups by calling:

- Your oncologist's office
- Your local hospital's social-service department
- The local chapter of a national disease-specific organization such as the Leukemia and Lymphoma Society, US TOO (prostate cancer), the National Alliance of Breast Cancer Organizations (breast cancer), and so on.
- Your local chapter of the Wellness Communities, Gilda's Club, or similar organization offering free psychosocial support
- National cancer organizations such as the American Cancer Society or the National Coalition for Cancer Survivorship
- Cancer Information Service of the National Cancer Institute (800-4-CANCER)

You can look in the Yellow Pages or White Pages under "cancer," "support groups," or "social-service organizations."

How do I deal with people who seem uncomfortable dealing with me?

Unfortunately, some people may feel uncomfortable dealing with you because of your illness. It may be that they want to help but don't know how. For these people, the simplest thing to do is to be direct. Tell them how they can help by saying something like "Thanks for calling (or writing). This is all new to me, and I appreciate your concern. Can we meet to talk over a cup of tea?" Or, "I'm not ready to talk, but could you call again in a week or two? May I call you?" Or, "I'm getting plenty of support from my family and my support group. I would really like to get together and talk about anything other than cancer."

Some friends may disappear in the face of your illness, even when you make it easy for them to keep in contact. You will likely experience grief over the loss of these friends, and the loss of your image of this friend. You may feel angry, lonely, or insecure; or you may feel guilty as if *you* have done something wrong. These people may have their own hang-ups about cancer; the problem is theirs, not yours. Try to focus on the important tasks at hand, and not on the disappointing response of some people.

Does everyone need support?

People are social beings. Even though talking with others doesn't change the facts of your illness, sharing your thoughts and feelings can change how you feel about what's happening. In an almost magical way, talking may bring you comfort, understanding, courage, or joy. Support from others can help you get the best medical care and minimize the pain, debility, and loss due to your illness.

The Rambo approach to cancer may get you through but accepting support will make the journey safer, easier, and less frightening.

Is there anything good about cancer?

Cancer is bad. But, good things can come out of the experience of surviving cancer. For you, getting on with business may be the order of the day. All you feel is relief (a good feeling) and gratitude. Or, you may feel your cancer is a wake-up call, and respond by changing important things about the way you see the world and act each day. In facing your mortality, you feel that you've learned how to live even better. Learning how to integrate the physical, emotional, social, and spiritual changes catalyzed by your diagnosis will help you live as fully as possible within the limits imposed by cancer treatment.

A cancer diagnosis encourages you to know both the fragility and hopes of life, and with this knowledge to live most fully.

6

Insights and Handles for Healthy Survivorship

Millions of people have traveled the cancer journey before you. The experience of these veteran survivors can provide insights and handles for helping you through these first few months after a cancer diagnosis. There is no way on earth to eliminate all the unpleasant emotions, discomforts, inconveniences, worries, strains, and uncertainties. However, you can learn ways to deal with the difficulties accompanying the evaluation and treatment of your cancer. You can learn techniques and philosophies that make the tough times easier.

A simple phrase or motto may help you through an unpleasant situation or mood more than all the sophisticated, caring discussion in the world. For example, you can investigate and analyze the series of problems that keep rocking your equilibrium, and you can struggle to understand your fluctuating moods. Or, you can simply say to yourself, "Cancer is a roller-coaster." You can spend fruitless hours trying to untangle tensions that are embroiled in complex family dynamics when you might be better served by the simple statement "Cancer is a family affair."

Handles make it easier to move from one place to another. The usefulness of each handle for surviving cancer depends as much on your personality, style, and particular situation as on the words themselves. Some of the following handles may become reliable mantras of comfort or inspiration throughout your evaluation and treatment. Others may not apply or be meaningful to you. Some may be helpful only under certain circumstances or at a few times during your treatment course. If a handle helps, use it. If it doesn't work for you, consider it again in a few weeks or months and, in the meantime, find others that work well now.

KNOWLEDGE IS POWER.
Sound information enables you to make wise decisions and to affect your life in positive ways.

A WISE TREATMENT CHOICE GIVES YOU THE BEST CHANCE OF THE BEST POSSIBLE OUTCOME.
Weigh your treatment options. Work together with your physicians to decide on a course of action. Once you've made a final treatment decision, take comfort and find confidence in the knowledge that what you are doing is expected to give you the best chance of the best overall outcome.

WEIGH APPLES AGAINST APPLES.
When you are making decisions regarding your care, make every effort to be logical and unemotional. Even more than you want to avoid conflict or confusion, you want the facts so that you can know your choices and weigh apples against apples. Even more than you want *easy* solutions, you want *effective* solutions (even if the solution involves a tougher course in the short run!).

BE TRUE TO YOURSELF.
Listen to your inner voice when you are presented with varied advice and facts about diet, doctors, treatments, and recovery techniques. Listen to your feelings to know how you are doing and what you need.

YOUR BODY IS WIRED TO HEAL ITSELF.
Your body is programmed to repair wounds, clear infections, and kill cancer cells. When normal cells are injured or destroyed in the process of getting rid of your cancer cells, your body natu-

rally sets in motion multiple mechanisms to recover. When you feel sick, remember that your body is hard at work doing what it is wired to do: heal.

TREATMENT DOESN'T HAVE TO GO PERFECTLY TO HAVE AN EXCELLENT OUTCOME.

Especially when your treatments are rigorous, you may have delays, setbacks and complications as part of what will prove to be an excellent outcome. Keep the big picture in mind, and do what you have to do to get through the ups and downs of treatment.

CANCER IS A ROLLER-COASTER.

Life after a cancer diagnosis is like a roller-coaster ride: good days and bad days; smooth weeks and weeks when nothing goes right; moments when you feel like you can handle all the stress and moments when you feel overwhelmed; hours when life looks richer and brighter than ever before, and hours when all the world appears gloomy; times when you are brimming with confidence and optimism, and times when you want to give up. When you are having a great day, enjoy it! On those rotten days, remember that it is okay to have a bad day, and that tomorrow may be better. As you go through treatment, you'll learn ways to prevent or minimize many of the problems that lend to the bad times.

LET GO OF THE "OLD NORMAL" WHILE GOING THROUGH TREATMENT.

For most survivors, it's impossible to make life feel the same as it did before their cancer diagnosis. Unexpected, unpleasant changes due to your cancer and its treatment occur and need to be integrated into your daily life. So, even when you are adjusting well, the rhythm of your life feels different than before. Change is a necessary condition of life, with or without illness. You are still you; you're just taking one of the sharper bends in your life. Routine and a sense of "normal" can be achieved again, even during treatment. But your "new normal" won't be the same as before.

CONTROL IS AN ILLUSION.

A cancer diagnosis makes you painfully aware of how little control you have over many important things, such as test results you can't change as well as anxiety-producing and time-consuming medical appointments, treatments, and discomforts. Your cancer did not create a loss of control; it revealed the lack of control that is part of life.

EXPECT STRONG EMOTIONS AND REACTIONS.

Handling a cancer diagnosis *well* does not mean handling it *calmly*; it means doing what you need to do to take care of the cancer while you work through your feelings, whatever they may be. The intensity of your emotions will lessen with time. Don't hesitate to have your doctor get you in touch with someone who can help determine if you would benefit from counseling.

NEGATIVE THOUGHTS ARE NORMAL AND DON'T CAUSE CANCER.

Thoughts of medical complications or death are a normal part of a healthy adjustment to your diagnosis of cancer. They reflect your fears and anxieties, not your wishes or predictions. If negative thoughts caused cancer, nobody would survive their diagnosis and we wouldn't have millions of cancer survivors in America today!

WHAT EMOTIONS YOU HAVE IS LESS IMPORTANT THAN WHAT YOU DO WITH THEM.

There are no "right" emotions to have. What you feel is what you feel. Unpleasant or painful emotions are the signal of a problem or the reaction to a problem. Fear, anxiety, anger, sadness, and other emotions become problems, themselves, when they keep you from taking care of your cancer or communicating with your family and friends. Share your thoughts and feelings with someone who cares and understands. Learn about the problems that trigger your unpleasant emotions as well as how to deal with the problems.

GRIEVING YOUR LOSSES IS HEALING.

A cancer diagnosis is accompanied by losses, some of which are temporary, some of which may be permanent. Grief is the human, healing reaction to loss. Expressed grief helps you accept and adapt to your loss so that you can move forward and recapture joy and excitement. Healing grief is temporary even when your loss is permanent. Over the next few weeks to months, expect to grieve for all the obvious losses such as a body part or function. You also may grieve the subtle losses such as your appetite, energy, or the comforting illusion of safety from illness.

CHANNEL YOUR ANGER.

Free-floating fury can hurt you by draining the energies you need for healing. You are the one who suffers when you direct your anger at people or events that can't be changed, or at people who can help you. Channel your anger toward overcoming the challenges of cancer treatment.

THE ONLY THING TO FEAR IS FEAR ITSELF.

Cancer is scary. Having courage doesn't mean being fearless; it means going for treatments and tests even when you feel afraid. Tame your fears by obtaining sound knowledge, finding and nourishing genuine hope, and taking effective action.

DO THE RGHT THING NO MATTER WHAT YOU MAY BE FEELING.

Your emotions may tempt you to go against your better judgment. Just as firefighters learn to enter smoke-filled fiery homes despite their normal and adaptive fear of flames, you can learn how to take the right steps (such as calling or visiting your doctors) to prevent problems even when you feel embarrassed, afraid, or angry. If it is too difficult to do the right thing or you are uncertain about what steps are best, get help from family, friends, or professionals.

KEEP PROBLEMS LIMITED TO WHAT THEY ARE TODAY.

When you have a problem such as pain, trouble sleeping, or nausea, try to deal with the problem *as it is* now. Avoid worrying about how it *might be* worse tomorrow. Anticipating tomorrow's possibilities may make today's problem more distressing than it would be otherwise, and doesn't help you deal with tomorrow when tomorrow comes.

AVOID THINGS THAT ARE NOT HELPING YOU.

If a news show or movie distresses you, turn it off. If someone's conversation makes you uncomfortable, tell him or her so (e.g.,

"I'd rather not talk about this topic now" or "This topic isn't good for me now"), change the subject, or leave. These calculated maneuvers do not mean that you are weak. They demonstrate your ability to recognize what is not good for your well-being and the strength to protect yourself from unnecessary burdens. Listen to your inner self to know what helps and what hurts you.

FOCUS ON WHAT YOU *CAN* DO NOW.

Regretting or worrying about the past is a waste of precious time, energy, and emotions because you can never change the past. Worrying about the future is also a waste. Fretting now won't prevent tomorrow's problems or make it easier to deal with them. Today's worrying just prolongs and deepens the pain associated with tomorrow's difficulties. And if the anticipated problem never occurs, you will have worried about a nonexistent problem. Focus on realistic ways to strengthen your physical, emotional, and spiritual health. Efforts toward real progress, no matter how small, are life enhancing.

IF YOU CAN DO IT YOURSELF, DO IT YOURSELF. IF YOU NEED HELP, GET HELP.

If you want help or expect help when you don't really need it, you slow down your recovery. If you refuse help when you really need it, you slow down your recovery, too. The key is in knowing what you can do on your own, and when it's best to get some help. If you're not sure, get help knowing when you need help.

AVOID MAKING COMPARISONS.

Looking to others for inspiration is not the same as comparing yourself to others, which can be defeating if you feel you don't measure up. Avoid *comparing* yourself to others who had or have cancer. Cancer survivorship is not a contest. It doesn't matter if someone else has a better or worse prognosis, or an easier or smoother course of treatment. It doesn't help you if another person adjusts better, worse, faster, or slower.

Avoid measuring yourself against your own expectations, too, such as how you "should" feel, physically or emotionally, or what you "should" be able to do at work, home, or in the doctor's office. Otherwise you might be very discouraged if you develop unexpected problems or complications, or if your experience is just not what you expected. Try to avoid comparing your current self to the way you were before treatment. Since your circumstances are now different, it would be like comparing apples and oranges. Instead of trying to get back to your old normal, see yourself as making progress toward a new normal.

THIS, TOO, SHALL PASS.

Nothing in life stays the same. If you are having a tough time, remember that no situation lasts forever. Your todays will become your yesterdays. Before you know it, you will talk about your tough times in the past tense.

CHOOSE YOUR BATTLES.

Don't waste your energy on little annoyances that are better left alone such as a dish that slips out of your hand and shatters on the floor. Save your energy for more important things, like getting through treatment. Go ahead and scream at the broken dish if this releases pent-up anger and frustration, doesn't hurt anyone else, and leaves you feeling better. This is different from getting all worked up about every little thing that goes wrong.

ACCEPTANCE IS LIKE A WAVE.

Even when changes in your life happen quickly, it may take you a long time before you understand and accept the changes and their consequences. You can know that you have cancer, and you can be taking all the right steps to treat it. Yet, it may be weeks or months before you totally accept the reality of your illness, if you ever *totally* accept it. Acceptance is a complicated process that occurs on many levels. Acceptance is like an ocean surf, ebbing and flowing, slowly making progress on the reef of disbelief or denial.

FIND AND NOURISH HOPE.

You can accept discouraging facts about your illness and still believe in the possibility of a good outcome. You can have genuine hope without expectations. You can hope for a long life or cure, physical comfort, or personal or spiritual growth. While there's life, there's hope.

HOPE IS DYNAMIC.

Your sense of hope fluctuates from day to day, even hour to hour, depending upon your circumstances. Focus on the factors under your control that can help you find and nourish hope. When possible, avoid the people and situations that pull down your hopefulness.

CANCER *VICTIMS* AND CANCER *SURVIVORS* ARE PEOPLE IN THE SAME SITUATION WITH DIFFERENT FRAMES OF MIND.

Choose to see yourself as a survivor or thriver or whatever other label helps you feel hopeful and empowered.

USE LIFE-ENHANCING LANGUAGE.

The way you think and talk about all the challenges and changes helps shape your perception of them. Listen to yourself and others, and choose to use life-enhancing language. Ask others to use life-enhancing language.

GOALS PROVIDE A FOOTING INTO THE FUTURE THAT ENHANCES YOUR TODAYS.

Set goals for yourself that you can work toward every day. Think of something that you want to get done, or need to get done. The goals can be as small as making a phone call, reading a newspaper, or getting through the next treatment. If you are able, focus on bigger or longer-term projects, too. Make the goals reasonable so you don't set yourself up to fail. When you accomplish a goal, enjoy the satisfaction of a job done.

THE BEST YOU CAN DO IS THE BEST YOU CAN DO.

Under the circumstances, you may not perform up to your usual standards for many tasks, and may not react to people or things the way you intend or would like to. Knowing what you want to do and doing it in real life are two completely different things. You are human, with human emotions and limitations. Nobody is perfect. Everyone has good days and bad days. Hopefully, you will learn as you go, finding new and better ways to handle life's challenges. Be kind to yourself.

CANCER IS A FAMILY AFFAIR.

Your diagnosis of cancer affects everyone involved in your life and everyone who cares about you. As trying as this situation may be for you, remember that it is hard for those who care about you, too.

YOU ARE NOT RESPONSIBLE FOR OTHERS' DIFFICULTIES DUE TO YOUR CANCER.

Your cancer is causing the problems, not *you*. You didn't try to get cancer so that you could cause others' distress. You are a package deal, and your presence in their lives means sharing the hard times as well as the happier times. It means giving as well as taking.

REQUEST AND ACCEPT HELP.

The Rambo approach to cancer may get you through, but finding and accepting help will allow a safer, easier, and less frightening journey. Accepting help gives others an opportunity to feel fulfilled.

DON'T REINVENT THE WHEEL.

Save yourself a lot of time and energy by learning shortcuts and insights from veterans who are positive role models. Use others' successes to inspire you ("If they can do it, it must be possible" or "I can do it, too").

LEARN HOW TO BE AN EFFECTIVE PATIENT.

Your physicians are trying to solve all your problems, little and big, with sensitivity and efficiency. When you make it easier for your doctors, they can do a better job for you.

DOCTOR VISITS ARE NOT SOCIAL SITUATIONS.

Come prepared for your doctor visits. Be honest about your symptoms or problems. Reporting symptoms is not complaining.

Wanting an understandable explanation is not wasting anyone's time.

BETTER TO BE SAFE THAN SORRY.
Between scheduled visits, if you are unsure about whether something needs to be reported or it can wait, call your doctors or nurses (even if it's 2 A.M.!) and let them decide if it needs attention now.

DOCTORS AND NURSES ARE NOT MIND READERS.
Share your concerns regarding your physical, psychological, emotional, or spiritual situations. Problems in any of these areas can affect your medical condition. Even when your doctors and nurses can't tend to them personally, they can get you the assistance you need. At the very least, it is best for you and your physicians if they are aware of all the factors affecting you. Also, inform your physicians if there is a problem with a physician or staff member. Give specific examples.

TRUST IS A HEALING FORCE.
Comfort and confidence flow in relationships built on mutual respect and trust. You need to be able to trust the people caring for you. If you have doubts about your physicians' abilities, judgments, or intentions, find doctors you can trust. Make it clear to your physicians the limits, if any, of how much information you want shared with your family. If you feel like you can't find any doctor you can trust, meet with a social worker or counselor who can help you establish a trusting relationship with a physician.

MOVE IT OR LOSE IT.
The human body was not intended to sit or lie still all the time. Talk with your physicians about safe movements, exercises, or physical therapy.

SLEEPING IS NOT WASTING TIME.
Getting adequate rest recharges your body's batteries and may speed and maximize your recovery. Remember that some cancers

and most treatments can cause fatigue that persists despite adequate rest.

FIND AND CREATE POCKETS OF HAPPINESS, AND ENJOY THEM.

You don't have to be free of all problems or assured of a smooth recovery before you can enjoy today. While you are enjoying a television show or telephone conversation, let yourself forget about your worries. Enjoy what you can when you can, even if it is just a momentary pleasure.

CELEBRATE THE MILESTONES.

Celebrate the end of your first treatment, your first checkup, getting through surgery, getting through the first phase of treatment (if you are scheduled for more than one type of treatment), your first set of scans, and so on. Plan something dependably fun and happy for your celebration such as crossing off the date on a calendar, calling a special friend, watching a favorite movie on television, or something else that feels good to mark the accomplishment.

LAUGH A LITTLE!

Take advantage of the comforting, empowering, and healing effects of laughter and happiness. As long as you don't jeopardize your treatments, it is healthy to escape being serious at times. Don't sit back and just wait to feel happy or amused; seek out and create joyful moments.

FIND YOUR BEST COPING METHODS.

You are a unique individual, and you need to find ways of coping that work well for you. A coping tool that worked well during past challenges probably will be useful now. Your illness is also an opportunity to learn new ways of coping. You may need to try various approaches in order to find one or two that work for you. What works best may change over the course of your treatments. A coping tool that is useful now may not work later. Conversely, another may be useless today but invaluable later.

Learn how to adapt your old coping skills to your current circumstances and how to add new techniques through participation in religious groups or cancer support groups, reading self-help literature, obtaining counseling, and talking with survivors of cancer and other illnesses.

LEARN HOW TO MINIMIZE THE DISCOMFORT DUE TO NEGATIVE THOUGHTS AND FEELINGS.
Find little phrases that help you handle the inconveniences, discomforts, fears, and disappointments of dealing with cancer. Here are a few examples of handles that may work:

- Think of each treatment as being one step closer to being better.
- When you have to undergo needle sticks or other uncomfortable procedures, instead of thinking about how much you have to *suffer,* think about what you have to *put up with.* Like taking out the garbage, it's no fun but it doesn't cause suffering.
- Try to see unpleasant changes due to your treatment (such as hair loss and low blood counts) as positive signs that the treatment is doing its job.
- Instead of referring to your treatments in derogatory terms such as "poison" or "toxin," talk in terms of the healing they offer. Think of them as tonics, providing a way to pain relief or cancer control. Treatments, no matter how toxic, are good for you because without them you would suffer and die.
- Avoid catastrophizing. For example, instead of saying, "This treatment is *too* hard," try "This treatment is *very* hard." Instead of thinking "I can't take this anymore," try "I need help dealing with this."

CANCER DOES NOT DEFINE YOU, UNLESS YOU LET IT.
Cancer does not define you; it is just one part of who you are. Sometimes, your illness will have to take center stage. Other times, you can let it fade into the background, even if only for a few days. If your cancer seems to be monopolizing everyone's attention even when you are willing and able (and wanting) to think about or do something non–cancer related, remind people that you are more than your cancer.

EMBRACING LIFE IS A CHOICE.

When life is not going the way you expected or planned, embrace the life you have, and live it.

LIFE IS GOOD, EVEN WHEN TIMES ARE TOUGH.

Life is good. Throughout your life, you'll have times that are easy or challenging, joyful or sad, smooth or rough, expected or surprising, frustrating or satisfying, empty or meaningful, full of passion or marked by indifference, energizing or debilitating. When times are tough due to your cancer treatments, remember that it wasn't life that changed, but your circumstances. Life is good.

Conclusion

___

You are a cancer patient. You didn't choose to be a cancer patient. Right now, not having cancer is not an option. The good news is that you are a cancer survivor with choices. You can decide about your evaluation and treatment, degree of involvement in your medical care, diet and exercise, and relationship with the members of your health-care team. You can choose how you relate to your friends and family, what you tell your children, how you spend your time, your level of optimism and sense of hope, and how you want to cope from day to day, even hour to hour. Knowing your realistic options, and how to choose wisely from among them, helps you get good care and live as fully as possible. My hope is that *Diagnosis: Cancer* has helped you see your choices about all aspects of your survival and has guided you toward making wise decisions *for you*.

These first few months are a transition period. As is true of any passage, it is stressful to suddenly face all the physical, social, and emotional changes accompanying a cancer diagnosis. My hope is that this book has made it more manageable. You've been introduced to information that can help you create a strong alliance with your health-care team. You've read about techniques and healing philosophies that have helped me and millions of other survivors deal with the challenges of survivorship.

This is just a start. To help translate ideas into action, the first appendix offers tips for being an effective patient. Later appendices include a glossary, and explanations of commonly ordered tests. The resource list will guide you and your family to invaluable information and support for handling anything and everything from finding a clinical trial or someone to help file insurance forms, to dealing with the twin challenges of raising children while undergoing cancer treatment, to understanding the unique concerns of the well person living with someone with cancer.

Having cancer is not easy. Learning about cancer and about how to cope with treatment can make your cancer experience easier, safer, and less frightening. Having cancer is not good. Learning about survivorship can free you to find some positive results from this unwanted situation. Sound knowledge, realistic hope, and effective action are the keys to Healthy Survivorship. The information and advice offered in *Diagnosis: Cancer* will help you integrate your new illness into your life in healing ways. There is life after a cancer diagnosis. Make it a good life.

As they say in poker, you can't choose your hand, but you can choose how you play it.

As they say in baseball, you can't choose your pitch, but you can choose how you hit it.

Appendix A

Tips for Being an Effective Patient

You get better care when you help your physicians and nurses care for you.

- Come prepared for your doctor visits. Call ahead if you are not sure if you are supposed to be fasting, bringing something, or taking or refraining from certain medications. Bring your list of questions and concerns.
- Be honest about your symptoms or problems. Reporting symptoms is not complaining. Wanting an understandable explanation of your illness or treatment is not "wasting" anyone's time.
- Trust your doctor. If you don't, find a doctor whom you do trust.
- Learn when you need to call the doctor's office, and when a noticeable change or a problem can wait. If you are unsure about calling (even if it's 2:00 A.M.), call and let the doctor or nurse decide if it needs attention. Better to be safe than sorry.
- Keep your physicians aware of your concerns regarding your physical, psychological, emotional, or spiritual situations.
- Inform your physicians if there is a problem with a physician or staff member. Give specific examples.
- Make clear to your physicians the limits, if any, of how much information you want shared with your family.
- Leave the doctor's office only *after* you are clear about all your instructions, prescriptions, appointments, tests, treatments, or follow-

up calls. Do not depend on the office or hospital to call and remind you.

- If you think you are supposed to be scheduled for a test and the office has not scheduled it or seems to know nothing about it, ask the staff to check with your doctor. Do not assume that the test was canceled or that you were in error.
- Make sure you get all your test results (blood work, scans, biopsies, etc.). Do NOT assume that no news is good news.
- If your doctors are running late because they are with other patients, remind yourself that your doctors are spending time with patients who need them. One day, that patient might be you and you'll be glad that your doctor takes the time needed to tend to you.

Appendix B

Glossary

Access: A connection between the outside of the body and the bloodstream.

Acute: Severe or having a rapid onset, and short-lived (not chronic).

Abdomen: Part of the body below the diaphragm; contains the stomach, kidneys, pancreas, intestines, and other organs.

Adenocarcinoma: Cancer that started in glandular tissue (e.g., breast, lung, thyroid, colon, pancreas).

Adjuvant chemotherapy: Chemotherapy given when there is no evidence by any tests for leftover cancer, but there is reason to be concerned that there still may be cancer cells in the body. It is given to decrease the chance of a recurrence.

Allograft: Bone marrow or stem-cell transplant in which the donor marrow is obtained from someone else and then given to the patient.

Allogeneic transplant: Allograft.

Alopecia: Hair loss.

Alternative cancer therapy: Unconventional cancer therapy used *instead* of conventional; cancer treatment that has not been proven scientifically to cure cancer; unorthodox cancer therapy.

Analgesic: Medicine that relieves pain.

Anaplastic cancer: A cancer whose cells, under the microscope, look very immature and different from the tissue in which it started.

Sometimes it is impossible to be sure where it started. These are usually faster-growing cancers.

Anemia: Low red blood cells or hemoglobin due to blood loss, blood destruction in the vessels, or impaired ability to make new blood.

Angiogram: X ray of blood vessels taken after injection of dye.

Antiangiogenesis agents: Drugs used to inhibit the growth and development of a tumor's blood supply.

Antibiotic: Drug used to fight bacterial infection.

Antiemetic: Antinausea; treatment to relieve nausea or vomiting.

Antioxidant: Agent that prevents a substance from combining with oxygen.

Anxiolytic: Medicine that counteracts or diminishes anxiety.

Apheresis: Technique of separating blood into components such as stem cells.

Apoptosis: Programmed cell death; cell death triggered by activation of certain genes.

Autograft: Bone marrow transplant in which the stem cells are taken from a patient and returned to the same patient after he or she receives the anticancer treatments.

Autologous transplant: Autograft.

Benign: Not cancer.

Biologic therapy (biologicals): Medicinal compounds that are prepared from living organisms and their products (e.g., vaccines, cytokines, serums, antitoxins).

Biopsy: Removal and examination under the microscope of a piece of tissue from a living person.

Bone marrow: Spongy substance in the center of bones; the place where blood is made.

Bone marrow transplant: Technique used to replace bone marrow destroyed by disease or cancer treatments; the donor cells are obtained from the bone marrow.

Breakthrough pain: Pain that occurs even though the patient is receiving medicine.

Cancer: A general term for over one hundred diseases characterized by abnormal and uncontrolled growth of cells. The mass, or tumor, can invade and destroy surrounding normal tissues. The cancer cells can spread through the blood or lymph system to start new cancers in other parts of the body.

Cancer of unknown primary: Cancer whose place of origin cannot be determined by any known means.

Carcinogen: Cancer-causing substance; substance that increases the risk of developing cancer in humans or lower animals.

Carcinoma: Cancer that begins in tissue that lines an organ or duct.

Cardiac: Pertaining to the heart.

Catheter: Tube (made of plastic, rubber, metal, or glass) passing into or through the body.

Cell: The unit structure of all living tissue.

Central line: A soft, hollow plastic tube with one tip sitting in a large vein near the heart and the other tip resting outside the body; a device for delivering fluids and medicines, and obtaining blood.

Chemotherapy: Treatment with anticancer drugs.

Chronic: Persisting for a long time.

Clinical trial: A carefully designed and executed investigation of the effects of treatments given to human subjects.

Clone: A group of cells all derived from a single cell.

Colony stimulating factor (CSF): A protein present in blood that stimulates the growth of certain white blood cells; includes granulocyte colony stimulating factor (G-CSF) and granulocyte macrophage colony stimulating factor (GM-CSF).

Combination chemotherapy: The use of two or more anticancer drugs.

Combination therapy: The use of two or more modes of treatment in combination, at the same time or one following the other.

Combined modality therapy: See **combination therapy.**

Complementary therapies: Unconventional therapies used *in addition to* conventional therapies.

Complication: Problem that may arise due to disease or treatment, and that may threaten the patient's health or life.

Comprehensive cancer center: Program delivering cancer care that fulfills criteria to be accredited by the National Cancer Institute; cancer center that provides standard cancer treatments, counseling, rehabilitation, and research and training facilities and staff.

Conventional cancer therapy: Treatment given to control or cure cancer that has been proven scientifically to be effective.

Cure: No evidence of cancer and the same life expectancy as if the person never had cancer; no evidence of cancer and no greater chance of developing cancer as if the person never had cancer.

Cyst: Sac containing fluid and/or solid material; usually benign, but can be malignant.

Debulking: Procedure to remove as much of the cancer as possible; reducing the "bulk" of the cancer.

Dendritic cells: Cells important in the body's immune response to specific antigens.

Diagnosis: The name of the illness.

Durable power of attorney: A legal document that allows you to appoint someone (an agent or proxy) to speak for you and make decisions for you when you are unable to do so yourself.

Erythropoietin (EPO): A protein that stimulates the production of red blood cells.

Estrogen: Female sex hormone.

Experimental treatment: Investigational treatment.

Gene: A piece of DNA in the chromosomes of cells that directs the proper functioning of the cell; the basic unit of heredity.

Gene therapy: Treatments being tested in research settings that work by changing the genetic makeup of cells.

Graft-versus-host disease (GVHD): Immune reaction between the transplanted cells and the patient's cells.

Growth factors: Chemicals that stimulate blood cells to grow.

Hepatic: Related to the liver.

Hormone: A substance from an organ or gland that travels through the blood to another part of the body, where it exerts its effect.

Immune system: A network of organs, cells, and substances distributed throughout the body to help protect the body against foreign invaders (or substances or cells interpreted to be foreign).

Immunotherapy: Treatment by stimulation of the body's immune defense system.

Implanted port: See **venous access port.**

Induction therapy: The initial treatment to eliminate or control cancer.

Informed consent: Competent and voluntary permission for a medical procedure, test, or treatment, given only after the subject understands the nature, risks, and alternatives available.

Infusion: Liquid substance introduced into the body via a vein for therapeutic purposes.

In situ cancer: Cancer that is confined and not invading normal tissues; cancer at a very early stage.

Interferons: Proteins produced by the body to help fight infection; they have been found to have some anticancer properties.

Interleukin: Substance derived from white blood cells that is involved in immune reactions to infection and cancer, and is being used in the treatment of certain types of cancer such as renal cell carcinoma.

Intramuscular: Into the muscle.

Intravenous: Through a vein.

Invasive cancer: Cancer that has invaded or spread into healthy tissue.

Investigational treatment: A drug or treatment that is under study; experimental treatment.

Kaposi's sarcoma: A type of skin cancer that can spread to other body parts and is usually seen in association with AIDS.

Late effects: Changes and problems that first appear months or years after completion of cancer treatment, and are due to the cancer or treatment.

Lesion: Abnormal area, may be benign or malignant.

Leukemia: Cancer that begins in the white blood cells in the bone marrow.

Living will: A written document that outlines how much you would want doctors to do to prolong your life (with medicines and machines) if you were critically ill with little hope of recovery; an advance directive that is not as powerful as the durable power of attorney.

Localized: Limited to the site of origin; no evidence of spread.

Lymph fluid: Clear fluid formed throughout the body, which flows in the lymph system, is filtered in the lymph nodes, and then is added to the blood.

Lymph nodes: Rounded bean-shaped organs that make some of the white blood cells (lymphocytes and monocytes) and filter the lymph fluid before it enters the blood; vary in size from a pinhead to the size of an olive; there are thousands of them throughout the body, the most obvious ones in the neck (cervical region), armpit (axillary region), and groin (inguinal region); may become a place to where cancer spreads.

Lymphatic system: A circulation system, like the blood system, that carries lymph throughout the body. Lymph is a colorless fluid that carries infection-fighting cells. The lymph organs include the lymph nodes, spleen, and thymus.

Lymphedema: Swelling due to blockage of lymphatic vessels.

Lymphoma: Cancer that begins in the lymphatic system, such as in a lymph node, the spleen, or the thymus gland.

Major depression: Mental state that has shifted for at least two weeks from a normal baseline to one that meets the criteria used to diagnose depression (depressed mood, decreased interest in activities or ability to experience pleasure, significant weight change, sleeping much more or less than normal, restlessness, being slowed down in thoughts and movements, fatigue, feelings of worthlessness, inappropriate sense of guilt, decreased ability to concentrate, indecisiveness, recurrent thoughts of death or suicide).

Malignant: Cancerous.

Metastasis (plural = metastases): Cancer cells that have spread from their original site through the blood or lymph and are now growing at another site.

Metastasize: To spread.

Monoclonal antibodies: Mass-produced antibodies that are all identical; sometimes used in the diagnosis or treatment of cancer; their usefulness for various cancers is being actively investigated.

Multiple myeloma: Cancer that begins in the plasma cells in the bone marrow.

Narcotic: Medicine that provides pain relief by depressing the central nervous system; opioid.

Neoplasm: Abnormal growth of tissue; may be benign or malignant.

Neuro: Pertaining to the nervous system.

Neutropenia: Low neutrophil (a type of white blood cell) count; this is associated with a high risk of infection.

Non-Hodgkin's lymphoma: A general term for a group of cancers of the lymphatic system that do not have the features of Hodgkin's lymphoma.

Nutritional support: Treatment aimed at preventing or treating malnutrition.

Oncologist: Doctor specializing in cancer diagnosis and treatment.

Oncology: The branch of medicine dealing with cancer.

Opioids: Narcotics; prescription medicine for moderate to severe pain.

Pathologist: Doctor specialized in diagnosing disease by looking at tissue directly, under the microscope, and with other technology.

Palliative: Treatment for comfort, not cure.

PDQ: "Physician Data Query": A frequently updated computerized list, provided by the National Cancer Institute, of ongoing clinical trials.

Platelet: Type of blood cell in the circulation; important in clotting (mechanism to stop bleeding).

Poorly differentiated cancer cells: Cancer cells that look immature and different from normal cells; the cancer tends to be faster-growing.

Port: See **venous access port**.

Precertification: Approval by a representative of your insurance company before you receive a specific medical service (or within a predetermined period of time).

Primary lesion: Original cancer; place where the cancer first arose.

Primary site: Place where the cancer first started.

Prognosis: Prediction of how well the patient will do.

Prosthesis (plural = prostheses): Artificial body part or aid.

Protocol: Description of the treatment steps (the "recipe").

Proxy: Someone with legal authority to act or make decisions for someone else.

Quackery: Promotion of a remedy that doesn't work or hasn't been proven to work.

Radioimmunotherapy: Anticancer therapy using monoclonal antibodies that are linked with a radioactive substance.

Radiation therapy: Treatment using radioactive substances.

Reactive depression: Situational depression; mental depression that follows severe life disappointment and usually resolves by itself.

Recurrence: Reappearance of the same cancer after a period when there was no evidence of cancer.

Regression: In psychology, a return to thinking and behavior more appropriate to a younger age.

Remission: Partial or complete shrinkage of cancer.

Renal: Pertaining to the kidney.

Residual disease (or cancer, or tumor): Remaining cancer.

Sarcoma: Cancer that begins in the soft tissue (muscles, nerves, tendons, blood vessels) or bones.

Sepsis: Infection in the blood.

Side effect: Unfavorable action or effect of a treatment.

Spleen: An organ in the left upper abdomen that is part of the lymph system. It helps to remove old red blood cells, produce white blood cells, and store blood.

Spontaneous remission: Disappearance of cancer without any treatment.

Staging: Evaluation to see how far the cancer has spread.

Standard treatment: Treatment that is recommended routinely; the safety and effectiveness are known.

Stem cell: Immature cell in the bone marrow and blood that gives rise to new bone marrow and blood cells.

Stem-cell transplant: Technique for replacing bone marrow destroyed by disease or cancer treatments; the cells for transplant are obtained from a vein in the arm of a donor.

Supportive therapy: Treatment given to help a patient feel better and regain health (treatment is not directed at cancer cells).

Therapeutic: Having healing properties.

Thrombopoietin: A protein that stimulates the production of platelets.

Tissue: Group of similar cells.

Titrate: To adjust the dose.

Tolerance: Progressive decrease in the effectiveness of a drug.

Total parenteral nutrition (TPN): Providing total calorie needs intravenously.

Tumor: An abnormal swelling or enlargement that may be either benign or malignant (cancerous).

Uterus: Womb (organ in which the unborn child grows).

Venous access device, vascular access device: A catheter or port that allows access to a major vein near the heart.

Venous access port: A device implanted under the skin that is used to obtain blood or give blood, fluids, or medicines.

Virus: A small germ that may cause infection; examples include Herpes, CMV (cytomegalovirus), and adenovirus.

Appendix C

Resources for the Newly Diagnosed Patient

NCI (NATIONAL CANCER INSTITUTE)
The Cancer Information Service (CIS) is a free service sponsored by the NCI. The CIS toll-free number, 800-4-CANCER, is answered by trained volunteers who are prepared to answer your questions about cancer or direct you to the place or person where you can get your answer. The NCI also offers a large number of informational booklets free of charge. After you are first diagnosed with cancer, you may want to request the booklet pertaining to your type of cancer entitled "What You Need to Know About Cancer." Two other booklets that are helpful in the beginning are "Taking Time" and "Facing Forward." You can request a list of all NCI's publications as well as the most recent printing of "PDQ" ("Physician's Data Query"). "PDQ" is a frequently updated summary of the work being done on your type of cancer. There is an edition for patients and an edition for physicians (you are welcome to both). You also can obtain the "PDQ" information summaries or other NCI information on the Internet by sending an e-mail message to cancernet@icicc.nci.nih.gov and writing the message "HELP" for a response in English, and "SPANISH" for a response in Spanish. Within minutes you should receive an e-mail listing of free publications that you then can order on line.

THE NATIONAL COALITION FOR CANCER SURVIVORSHIP (NCCS)
The National Coalition for Cancer Survivorship is the only survivor-led advocacy organization working exclusively on behalf of people with all

types of cancer and their families. NCCS has a strong voice on Capitol Hill and is a reliable source for information, programs, and resources on cancer survivorship. Their Web site includes CanSearch, an on-line tour guide designed to assist you with finding credible on-line cancer information and resources. They provide exceptional booklets such as "You Have a Right to Be Hopeful" and "Teamwork."   You can also request free of charge The Cancer Survival Toolbox™, an award-winning audio program that teaches skills that can help people with cancer meet the challenges of their illness.

> National Coalition for Cancer Survivorship
> www.canceradvocacy.org
> 1010 Wayne Avenue, 5th Floor
> Silver Spring, Maryland 20910
> 301-650-8868

THE AMERICAN CANCER SOCIETY (ACS)

The American Cancer Society has national and local offices. You can obtain the telephone number of the local office from your oncologist or the Yellow Pages. They have trained volunteers, many of whom have dealt with cancer personally, to answer questions. The ACS usually can provide information and referrals such as lists of local oncologists, support groups, and supply stores. The ACS offers a wide variety of services that provide information, comfort, and support. "Reach to Recovery" and "Look Good . . . Feel Better" are two popular programs. The Cancer Survivors Network (CSN) is a virtual support group that you join either with a phone call or on the Internet (www.acscsn.org). At your convenience, and from the privacy of your home, you can have live, private chats with other survivors of your choosing; find other survivors or family caregivers like yourself; share your experiences, thoughts, wisdom, inspirational messages; start or join virtual support communities of people who share your concerns and interests; post or find information about resources.

SOCIAL SERVICES

The social-services department of your local hospital is usually well versed in all the services available in your community (support groups, local supply stores, local support services, local treatment facilities).

THE OFFICE OF YOUR ONCOLOGIST

Your oncologist's staff is familiar with most of the needs and problems that you will have, as well as services available in the local community.

Appendix D

———

Sample Medication list

Week of _____

Time	MEDICINE	Dose	Sun	Mon	Tue	Wed	Thu	Fri	Sat

Appendix E

———

Explanation of Commonly Ordered Tests

Tests play an important role in the diagnosis and treatment of cancer because they help your doctors to:

- Determine the extent of your cancer at the time of your original diagnosis
- Uncover any coexisting or related problems at the time of your original diagnosis
- Establish a baseline for your follow-up studies
- Monitor the response of your cancer to the therapy
- Identify and evaluate any complications that may develop during treatment

There are seven basic categories of tests:

- Blood tests
- Urine tests
- Stool tests
- X-ray studies
- Nuclear scanning studies
- Ultrasound studies
- Endoscopy procedures

The risks (potential complications) for each test may vary from patient to patient depending on

- which technique is used to perform the test;
- the experience of the people administering and interpreting the test;
- your medical condition.

Invasive tests are riskier than noninvasive tests. Tests that require more X-ray exposure carry more long-term risk than tests that require less X-ray exposure. Contrast (dye that is ingested, injected, or given by enema) can cause problems in susceptible people.

When deciding which tests to order, your doctors weigh the risk, inconvenience, and expense of each test against the benefit of the information gained. If your doctor recommends a test and you decline it (or modify the test process in some way), you may be taking a risk with your health since the information provided by the test is felt to be valuable in making decisions about your care.

The time required for performing the test will vary depending on

- the speed of the specific equipment used;
- your medical condition (for example, how easy it is to find a vein for injection, or how well you can hold still or hold a deep breath);
- the quality of the pictures or samples (for example, if the pictures are fuzzy, they will have to be retaken; if the biopsy specimen is too small, it will have to be redone).

An estimate of the time it takes to undergo a test does not include the time you wait in the reception area, the time it takes to set up the test, or any recovery time required following completion of the test.

When you schedule a test, be sure that you are clear about

- the time when you are supposed to arrive for your test;
- the place where you are supposed to go for your test;
- any dietary restrictions prior to the test;
- any special medication that is supposed to be taken or preparation that is supposed to be completed prior to the test;
- whether you are supposed to take all your regular medicines on the day of your test;
- whether or not you will need someone to accompany you to or from the test.

Make sure the people doing the test are aware if you have

- a history of asthma or allergies, especially allergies to iodine or latex;
- any chance of being pregnant;
- a bleeding disorder;
- a tendency toward claustrophobia or fear of needle sticks.

The results of your test are sent to the doctor who ordered the test (usually your oncologist), who will then review the results with you. Expect a delay between the completion of a test and the availability of a final report. Preliminary reports are sometimes provided by your doctor's office. You can ask the people doing the test how long it usually takes for your doctors to get the final results. Do not assume that no news is good news. If you have not heard the results of your test by the time they should have been available, have the doctor's office review the results with you.

Try not to let your imagination read anything into the facial expressions or idle banter of the technicians performing your test. Also, don't panic if they request that you repeat or add additional tests. Many times the news is good.

TYPES OF TESTS

Blood Tests

Phlebotomists (technicians who draw blood) wear gloves to protect themselves from any communicable infections that may be carried in their patients. There is no risk to you of acquiring a blood-borne infection when blood is taken from you with sterile equipment.

If you tend to faint when blood is drawn, let the phlebotomist know this before he or she begins. When blood is drawn from a vein, the phlebotomist will probably first place a tourniquet around your arm. Let the phlebotomist know if your arm or hand is uncomfortable or becoming numb, or if you feel faint.

Before the phlebotomist begins, be sure to point out if you have an I.V., central line, or fistula (for kidney dialysis). When possible, blood should not be drawn from the arm on the same side as a mastectomy or axillary lymph node dissection.

After the blood specimen is obtained, apply pressure to the puncture site until it stops bleeding. Let the phlebotomist know if the puncture site won't stop bleeding.

X Rays

X-ray studies can be as simple as a plain chest X ray, which takes one minute and exposes you to relatively little irradiation, or as complicated as an **angiogram**, which requires placing a catheter into a major artery and injecting dye before taking the X-ray pictures.

The contrast material used with some X-ray studies may interfere with the ability to perform other tests. (For example, barium given for an X ray of the colon may interfere with an ultrasound done soon afterward.) Usually your tests are prescribed in the proper order. As backup, it doesn't hurt to mention all the tests you are supposed to have to the people scheduling your X rays with contrast.

If there is any chance you are pregnant, let your doctors and the technicians know. When contrast is needed for the test, be sure to notify your doctor if you

- take a "beta-blocker," a type of medicine commonly prescribed for high blood pressure or heart disease (your doctor or pharmacist can tell you if any of your medicines are beta-blockers);
- have asthma or heart disease;
- have ever had an allergic reaction to contrast material.

If any of the above conditions apply, your doctors may:

- Order an alternative test that doesn't use contrast
- Prescribe antiallergy medications such as Benadryl and/or steroids prior to the test

You will need to remove all metal objects, such as necklaces, watches, metal belt buckles, and pins, before X rays because they cast shadows that can block visualization of important structures.

Let the technicians know if you develop any symptoms during or after the test, especially if you notice itching, rash, wheezing, shortness of breath, nausea, light-headedness, heart palpitations, or chest pain.

If contrast is used, you may be asked to drink a lot of fluids afterward to help flush out the contrast and prevent kidney problems.

Nuclear Scanning
To perform a nuclear scan, a substance that gives off radiation (a radionuclide) is administered, after which scans are done to measure the amount of radiation of the target organ(s). Only minimal radiation exposure occurs, and you do not pose any significant risk to others after the test (your body rids itself of the tracer amount of radioactivity in six to twenty-four hours). You may be asked to drink extra fluids after the

test to help flush the radioactive substance out of your system (in your urine). You may also be asked to flush the toilet several times after you void to wash away the radionuclide-containing urine.

Be sure to notify your doctors and the technicians performing the test if:

- You may be pregnant
- You are nursing a baby
- You have had any recent nuclear scans (the previous study could interfere with the interpretation of the current test)
- You have a tendency toward claustrophobia
- You have trouble lying still (e.g., because of pain)

Ultrasound Tests

Ultrasound tests use harmless sound waves to image certain body areas such as the **abdomen**, pelvis, heart, and pregnant uterus. There is no radiation risk involved. To perform the test, first gel is placed on the skin overlying the area to be evaluated. Then a transducer, which looks like a wand or a microphone, is placed on the gel and slowly slid along your skin. You will have to lie still at times, and you may have to hold your breath periodically. If the pelvis is being imaged, you will probably need to have a full bladder. You will be asked to fast (not eat) if the gallbladder is being evaluated. Air bubbles can interfere with ultrasound, so do not drink any carbonated drinks prior to your test.

(Average time: thirty minutes for the abdomen, fifteen minutes for the breast)

Endoscopy Procedures

Advances in fiber optics have allowed the visualization of many internal structures, such as the esophagus, stomach, colon, airways, urinary system, and joints. Oftentimes, biopsies can be obtained, and sometimes therapeutic maneuvers (such as stopping a bleeding ulcer) can be accomplished through the fiber-optic equipment.

Endoscopic procedures are done by specialists after obtaining written informed consent. If you are sedated during the procedure, you will probably need to have someone else take you home after the test.

Specific Tests

Angiogram = arteriogram = contrast vascular study (X ray)

After contrast material is injected into an artery, pictures of blood vessels can be taken. Doctors gain information about the shape, size, and distribution of blood vessels. This helps define the blood supply to a tumor, and indicates when there is disease of the blood vessels (such as a blood clot or hardening of the arteries).

Using gentle sedation and local anesthesia, a catheter (thin plastic tube) is inserted into an artery. Usually the large artery in the groin is used as the entry site, although occasionally another artery is used. Dye is injected into an artery supplying the area to be studied, and rapid-sequence X rays are then taken. There is minimal discomfort other than having to lie still on a hard table. Angiography is a higher-risk study, but is still relatively safe in skilled hands. (Average time: 90 minutes)

cerebral angiogram = picture of vessels to the brain
coronary angiogram = picture of vessels to the heart
pulmonary angiogram = picture of vessels to the lung
renal angiogram = picture of vessels to the kidney
visceral angiogram = picture of vessels to the organs in the abdomen

Barium Enema = BE (X ray)

This is an X ray of the colon and rectum. Your doctors may prescribe medicines to clean out the colon prior to the X ray. For the test, barium is given by enema into the rectum, where it outlines the inner surface of the colon and rectum. If an air-contrast barium enema is ordered, air is introduced into the rectum after the barium.

You may feel distended and uncomfortable as you hold the barium and air in your colon while the X rays are taken. If you feel weak and tired from the preparation or test, it is advised that you have someone take you for your test. The radiologist or your doctor may prescribe laxatives for you to take after the test to clear the barium from your colon. (Average time: twenty to forty minutes)

Barium Swallow (X ray)

This is an X ray of the pharynx (throat) and esophagus. A barium-containing liquid, and sometimes a barium-containing wafer, is swallowed. X rays are taken while you are swallowing, to show the contractions of the esophagus, as well as outline the inner surface of the pharynx and esophagus. Pictures may be taken while you are in different positions. Some people find the taste of the barium solution unpleasant. It is important to clear the barium from your system after the test; laxatives may be prescribed. Your stools will be white at first and then return to your normal color when the barium is cleared. (Average time: five to twenty minutes)

Bone Marrow Biopsy (blood test)

This is a test to obtain a sample of bone marrow for analysis. The sample is usually obtained from the marrow in your hip or your sternum (breast-bone). If you tend to get anxious, you may request a mild relaxant, although you will have to have someone else drive you home if you do.

While you are lying on an exam table or hospital bed, the skin and bone are made numb using local anesthetic (you may have some brief burning or pain as the numbing medicine is administered). When the area is numb, a special needle is then put into the bone and a sample of the marrow is withdrawn. There is the sensation of painless pressure as the needle is pushed through the bone into the marrow. There is pain for a second or two as the marrow is removed, and you may be sore at the site of the biopsy for a few days. Mild pain relievers may be prescribed. The entire procedure takes ten to twenty minutes. Notify your doctor if you develop fever or increasing pain, redness, or swelling at the puncture site.

Bone Scan (nuclear scan)

A bone scan uses a small amount of injected radioactive substance to picture all the bones in your body. Abnormalities show up as areas of increased (hot spots) or decreased radioactivity. Hot spots can be due to cancer, arthritis, a fracture, or other nonmalignant diseases. Bone abnormalities can show up on a bone scan months before they show up on a plain X ray of the bone.

You receive an injection in your vein containing the radioactive substance one and one-half to two and one-half hours prior to the scan, during which time you may be asked to drink a lot of water. Some people find it uncomfortable to lie still on the hard scanner table for the thirty to sixty minutes it takes to do the scan. The scanner is a big machine that lies inches away from you; tell your doctors and the technicians if you tend to have claustrophobia.

CT Scan = CAT Scan = Computerized Axial Tomography = Computed Tomography (X ray)

This is a sophisticated X ray that shows cross-sectional views of the area pictured. In many cases, CT scans are used instead of surgery to help stage and follow cancer (see chapter 1). In order to improve the visibility of certain tissues and organs, you may be asked to drink some contrast before being scanned (these solutions aren't tasty, but they've improved over the years). Dye may be injected into a vein during the test to help the radiologist distinguish the different organs and structures. You may be asked to hold your breath for a few moments while some of the X rays are taken. Areas of your body may be scanned without contrast, and then scanned again after contrast is given. Sometimes the preliminary pictures prompt the need for repeating the scan with thinner slices (this doesn't necessarily mean there is a problem; the preliminary pictures may not visualize an important area well).

You will be alone in the room during the X rays, but you will be able to talk with the technicians throughout the test via a two-way intercom. People with a tendency toward claustrophobia may feel anxious during this test. Medication can be given to help this anxiety, so discuss this with your doctor. Some people find it uncomfortable to lie still in one position for the duration of the test. It takes approximately thirty minutes to do one scan of the head, chest, abdomen, or limb. With the newer helical (spiral) scanners, the scan is much faster and you only need to hold your breath one to three times.

Cystogram = Voiding Cystography = Cystourethrography (X ray)

This is a picture of your urinary bladder. Dye is introduced into your bladder through a urinary catheter. You may find it uncomfortable for a few seconds when the catheter is placed in your bladder, and while you are holding a full bladder as the pictures are taken. The testicles can be shielded from the radiation; ovaries cannot be shielded without impairing the view of the bladder. Let your doctors know if you are having any urinary difficulties (burning, pain, difficulty voiding, blood in the urine) after the test. (Average time: fifteen to thirty minutes)

Flow Cytometry

This is a specialized test done on blood or tissue samples. This test identifies specific markers on, and in, small numbers of cancer cells. Most often used for cases of blood cancer (leukemia and lymphoma), it can help make a definite diagnosis and sometimes provides information that is useful in making a prognosis.

Gallium Scan (nuclear scan)

This scan uses tracer amounts of gallium to look for areas of inflammation or dividing cells (infections, abscesses, and benign and malignant tumors). Not all cancer picks up gallium. You do not pose any risk to others because of the tiny amount of radioactive tracer in your system.

First, you receive one injection containing the radioactive tracer in a vein in your arm. Four to six hours later a total-body scan may be done. Twenty-four hours after the injection, and again forty-eight hours after the injection, you lie still on a hard table as the scanner takes the pictures. Each scan takes thirty to sixty minutes.

Intravenous Pyelogram = IVP = Excretory Urography (X ray)
This is an X ray of the kidneys, ureters, and bladder. You may be given a cathartic to clean out the colon prior to the test. At the beginning of the test, dye is injected into your vein, after which X rays are taken of your kidneys as the dye is excreted. If your kidney function is normal, multiple X rays will be taken over twenty to thirty minutes. If there are kidney problems, X rays may need to be taken periodically for a few hours. You may be requested to return for more X rays later in the day or the next day. After the test, drinking lots of fluids will help prevent dehydration related to fasting and the preparation for the test.

Make sure your doctors, the radiologist, and the technicians know if you:

• Have had an allergic reaction to contrast in the past
• Are dehydrated (haven't been able to keep fluids down; have had significant diarrhea)
• Have kidney disease, asthma, or heart disease
• Have multiple myeloma
• Have had a barium study recently

Liver-Spleen Scan (nuclear scan)
This is a picture of your liver and spleen that can detect defects greater than two centimeters in diameter. First, you receive an injection containing the radioactive tracer in a vein in your arm. Twenty to thirty minutes later, you lie still on a hard table for twenty to thirty minutes as the scanner makes the picture.

Lumbar Puncture = Spinal Tap
This is a simple procedure to obtain spinal fluid for analysis. After an area in your back is made numb with local anesthetic, a needle is inserted through the skin between two bones of the spinal column and into the

fluid-filled space of the spine. If you have a lot of curvature or arthritis, this procedure is sometimes done with X-ray guidance. You have to hold still during the test. It is usually painless, taking five to ten minutes. A few people will complain of a headache afterward, a problem that is decreased by lying flat for up to twelve hours after the test. Notify your doctors if, at any time, you have headache, pain or drainage at the injection site, trouble voiding, or numbness, tingling, or difficulty moving any extremity.

Mammogram (X ray)

A mammogram is a picture of the breast using low-dose X rays and high-speed film (the radiation exposure is very small). It is used to screen for breast cancers too small to be felt, and to evaluate lumps or skin changes of the breast. A mammogram is not foolproof: If a lump is suspicious, it should be biopsied even when the mammogram is normal. Although breast augmentation may interfere with total visualization of the breast, mammography still has value in these patients.

Before your mammogram, remove any jewelry around the neck and wash off any talc powder (which can cause suspicious-appearing spots on the picture). For the test, you stand in front of a small table on which your uncovered breast is placed. A special plate then flattens the breast against the table, and the X ray is taken. Large-breasted women sometimes find the breast compression uncomfortable. Small-breasted women sometimes find leaning their rib cage against the table uncomfortable. However, the test takes only five to ten minutes.

MRI Scan = NMR Scan = Magnetic Resonance Imaging Scan

This is an imaging technique that uses a magnetic field and radio waves instead of X rays. There are many advantages of MRI over CT, including:

- The pictures are quite detailed.
- Dye is used less frequently.
- Serial studies can be done without additional risk to the patient.

There are some disadvantages, too, including:

- Some MRI scanners feel more enclosed than CT scanners and cause significant anxiety in patients with a tendency toward claustrophobia (medication can be given to minimize this anxiety).
- MRI scans take longer to do than CT scans.

- MRI scans cannot be done on patients who have pacemakers or surgical clips for cerebral aneurysms.
- Expense

It is crucial that you hold perfectly still (which some people find uncomfortable) during the test. Because of the loud tapping sound, you might want to request earplugs to minimize the discomfort due to this noise. Be sure to remove all metal objects prior to your scan, because they will possibly interfere with the test and they can be dangerous because the magnet can pull them like a projectile. In particular, remove watches, dental bridges, jewelry, hair clips, belt buckles, and credit cards. Note that the scanner can erase the computer strip on your credit cards (and make them unusable) and can damage watches.

Newer MRI scanners include some with a more open design to allow testing of patients who are claustrophobic, obese, or in need of monitoring or supportive equipment. MRI-guided biopsies and procedures can be done. (Average time: thirty minutes for a scan of the head, sixty minutes for other scans)

Myelogram = Myelography (X ray)
This is an X-ray test to show the spinal cord. Dye is injected into the spinal fluid (see *lumbar puncture* in this Appendix), after which you lie prone on a table which is tilted at various angles to allow the dye to flow around to all parts of the spinal cord. X rays are taken in different positions. There may be discomfort associated with the spinal tap. A few people develop a headache after the procedure. If a water-soluble contrast is going to be used, be sure your doctors and the radiologist know which medicines you are taking. You will have to remain lying down or semi-erect for a while after the test is completed. Frequently, a CT scan is done after the myelogram. (Average time: forty-five minutes for one section of the spine, longer if the entire spine is to be evaluated)

Plain Radiography = Plain X ray = Plain Film = X ray
This is a standard X ray. It involves low-dose radiation exposure and only takes a few minutes. It is generally painless, although some positioning requirements may cause discomfort.

Positron Emission Tomography = PET Scan (nuclear scan)
This is a technique that combines the benefits of nuclear and CT studies. Besides providing some pictures of organ anatomy (shape and size),

the scans provide information about organ function. In cancer patients, PET scans provide information about the effects of cancer treatment on malignant tissue and the reaction of the surrounding normal tissue.

There are still a number of important limitations to this technique, including:

- High expense
- Limited availability (a cyclotron, chemical facilities, specialized computer equipment, and a group of highly specialized people are required to perform and interpret the test)

In preparation for a PET scan, avoid caffeine, alcohol, or tobacco for at least twenty-four hours. For comfort, empty your bladder just before the test. Usually two intravenous lines are placed before the scan. After the test, drinking fluids will help wash the radionuclide from your system. (Average time: sixty to ninety minutes)

UGI = Upper GI = Upper Gastrointestinal Series (X ray)

This is an X ray of the stomach. A contrast-containing solution is swallowed, during and after which X rays are taken. In an air-contrast upper GI study, you will be asked to swallow rapidly some carbonated powder that forms gas in the stomach. If additional pictures are taken after the contrast passes from the stomach into the small bowel (intestines), the additional X rays are called a "small bowel follow-through (SBFT)." You will lie on a special table that tilts. You may feel bloated or mildy nauseated during the test. If Gastrografin is used as contrast, you may have diarrhea after the test. If a different contrast is used, you may be given a laxative afterward to help eliminate the dye. Your stools should return to normal color after you expel the dye. (Average time: thirty to sixty minutes for a UGI, up to five hours for an SBFT)

Appendix F

Medical Abbreviations

Here is a list of frequently used abbreviations that you may see on your prescriptions, instructions, or insurance forms. Whenever you are not sure about an abbreviation, check with your doctor's office or your pharmacist.

a.c.	=	before meals
ad. lib.	=	as desired, as much as you want
b.i.d.	=	b.d. = two times a day (check if they want you to take the medicine or treatment every twelve hours, or just any two times during the day)
aa	=	a = of each
c.	=	with
ext.	=	extract
fl	=	fluid
gtt	=	a drop
gtts	=	drops
hgb	=	hemoglobin (related to red-blood-cell count)
h.s.	=	at bedtime
I.M.	=	intramuscular = in the muscle
I.V.	=	intravenous = in the vein
kg	=	kilogram
N.P.O.	=	nothing by mouth = fasting
p.c.	=	after meals

p.o.   = per os = given by mouth
p.r.n. = as needed (for example, "every six hours p.r.n." means
           that you can take the medicine as often as every six
           hours, but you would only take the medicine if you
           needed it)
q.   = every (for example, "Q. 8 hrs" means every eight hours)
q.a.m. = every morning
q.d.   = every day
q.h.   = every hour
q.h.s. = every evening
q.i.d. = four times a day
q.o.d. = every other day
s   = without
sig   = write = let it be labeled
suppos. = suppository
t.i.d. = three times a day

Index

Americans with Disabilities Act, 153
analgesics, 110, 223
anaplastic cancer, 223–24
anemia, 69, 127, 224
anger, 169–70, 210
angiogenesis inhibitors, 41, 224
angiograms, 224, 237, 238–39
antiangiogenesis agents, 41, 224
antibiotics, 34, 224
antibodies, monoclonal, 35–36, 228
anticipation, negative, 210
antidepressant medications, 167, 169
antiemetic, 69, 224
antigen-presenting cells (APC), 70
antioxidants, 83–85, 224
anxiety:
    diagnosis and, 162–63
    medical information and, 158
    pain and, 107–8, 114–15
    over past and future, 170–72, 211
    second opinions and, 58
    over treatment choice, 67, 171
    over treatment risks, 55
anxiolytics, 171, 224
apheresis, 38, 224
apoptosis, 12, 224
arteriogram, 238–39
asbestos, 14
Association for Applied and Therapeutic
        Humor, 87
attitude, positive, 181–85
autologous transplants (autografts), 38,
        224
Ayurvedic medicine, 73

barium enema (BE), 237, 239
barium swallow, 239
Becky and the Worry Cup (Harpham), 201
"benign," 8, 224
benzene, 14
beta-blocker, 237
beta-carotene, 83
bioelectromagnetics, 73
biofeedback, 81, 114

biologic therapy (biologicals), 32, 35, 73,
        224
biopsies, 6, 22, 224, 238
    bone marrow, 239
bladder, X rays of, 241
blame, 175–76, 177
bleeding, 89
blood, drawing of, 93
Blood and Marrow Transplant Newsletter,
        145
blood protein levels, 71
blood tests, 93, 236
    bone marrow biopsy, 239
blood vessels, cancer of, 7
bone marrow, 6–7, 224
    biopsies of, 240
    harvest of, 37
    plasma cells in, 7
    transplants, 37, 145–46, 224
bone scan, 240
bones, cancer of, 7
brachytherapy, 33
breakthrough pain, 112, 224
breast cancer, 5, 6, 35
Broviac central venous catheters, 96–97
bruising, 89
Burzynski's antineoplastons, 73

cancer:
    aggravating factors in, 14
    AIDS and, 12, 17–18
    anaplastic, 223–24
    causation, 14–17
    contagiousness and, 11
    defined, 4–5, 224
    depression and, 165–69
    development of, 11–13
    diet as factor in, 14, 17; *see also* nutrition
    doctors specializing in, *see* oncologists
    emotional reactions to, 161–73, 209,
        217
    environmental/lifestyle role in, 14
    family history of, 16
    fear and, 5, 114, 210